CONTENTS

PALEO DIET FOR BEGINNERS

KETO DIET FOR BEGINNERS

PALEO DIET
FOR BEGINNERS

Ultimate Guide for Rapid Weight Loss

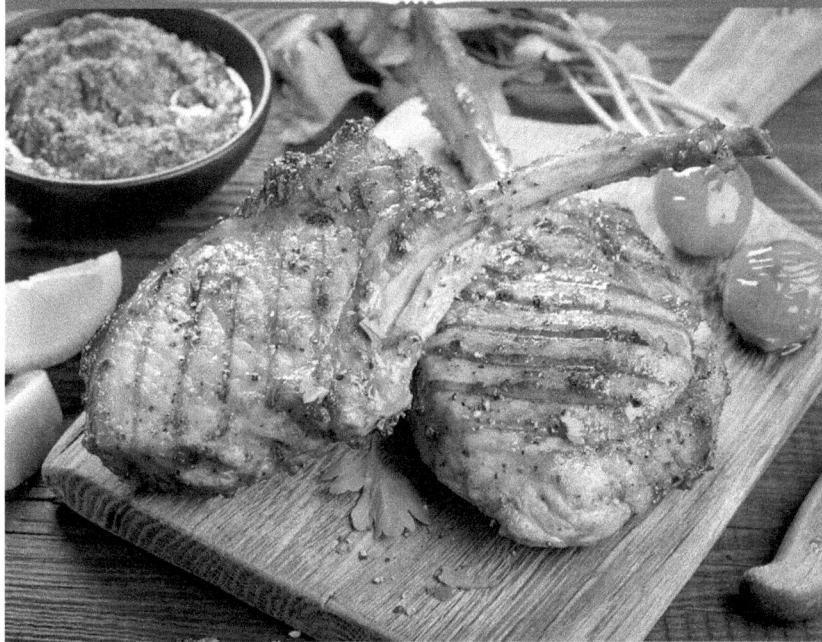

Cindy Chen

INTRODUCTION TO THE PALEO DIET

What Is the Paleo diet?

The Paleo diet is considered a primal or "caveman" diet, because it focuses on food options that were around during ancient times, before farming and the cultivation of crops was developed.

Principles of the Paleo Diet

Before you begin adapting to the paleo way of eating, it's important to understand the principles of the reasoning behind the food choices and meal options available. There are some basics to become familiar with when you begin, to have a good foundation of understanding:

- This diet includes foods in their most natural, unprocessed state, without any preservatives or additives. In adhering to these parameters, you'll avoid hidden sugars, artificial sweeteners, and over-processed boxed and packaged foods.
- Plant-based options are entirely fresh or frozen, often avoiding canned as an option, due to the high level of

preservatives often included. Dried fruit and vegetable chips are a great option, though best as homemade.

- Foods associated with cultivation, such as grains, legumes, and beans are avoided, as they do not fit within the primal options of food that paleo includes. Since farming wasn't developed during ancient primal times, these foods are generally avoided.

- High carbohydrate foods like rice, grains, and pasta are skipped, and instead, the focus is on root vegetables and organic fruits for a better carb option. Paleo doesn't specifically limit or avoid carbohydrates, though it focuses on natural, organic foods that contain high-quality carbs, which make a significant impact on the nutritional value of your meals.

- Nuts and seeds are strong staples in the paleo diet and cater to many variations of this way of eating, including plant-based and low carb. They are best consumed in their natural form, without any sugar, sodium, or flavoring added.

- All meat, specifically lean cuts of beef, pork, chicken, and turkey, are included in the paleo diet. Fish is an excellent option for including healthy fats, protein, and calcium. Game meats such as venison, are also a welcome inclusion in this way of eating.

- Dairy is not generally included, especially in strict Paleo diets; however, some may include small amounts.

Consider the types of foods our ancestors had access to thousands of years ago, before farming, cultivation, and processing. During those times, you ate what you could find or forage for, and the animals you hunted. This was a simple and effective way of feeding yourself, family, and community. Food wasn't necessarily cooked or prepared in any way, but enjoyed in its complete and natural state, whether it was raw meat, fish, berries, root vegetables, leaves, insects and other forms of animals and vegetation, depending on the region and the climate.

The Benefits of Adapting to the Paleo Way of Eating

What are the advantages of following a Paleo diet? There are plenty of reasons to adapt to this way of eating, and understanding the specific benefits can be a major reason to make the change. The impact of the paleo method will have a significant effect on your physical and mental health. The following advantages are common in many people who adapt to the paleo method:

Weight Loss

One of the most common reasons for adhering to the paleo diet is weight loss, and the ability to maintain a healthy weight for the long-term. The high fiber and nutrient content ensure your body receives a balanced diet complete with just the right amounts of natural sugar, sodium, and healthy fats, without excessive amounts of any content. The paleo diet's carb content tends to range from low to moderate, depending on the types of vegetables and fruits chosen for meal preparation and planning. Studies conducted on the results of participants following a paleo diet indicate consist of weight loss with significant improvement within a short period. Consistent weight loss results are a positive sign of the effects that the Paleo diet has on your body and metabolic function in general.

Muscle Gain and Healthier Bones

If losing muscle density is a concern, paleo will increase and keep your bones and muscles strong and healthy for the duration of your lifetime. In addition to containing adequate levels of vitamin C, A, and E, which aid in the absorption of vitamin D, your body will have sufficient amounts of calcium and protein. Together, these nutrients ensure your bones and cartilage remain healthy and strong, preventing deterioration of the spine and vertebrae as you age. Following the elements of Paleo can help prevent osteoporosis and arthritis, among other conditions that are related to age and degeneration.

A Better Night's Rest

Insomnia will soon become a thing of the past, as you experience an improved quality of sleep and more of it. You'll toss and turn less and be able to "crash" sooner and feel refreshed in the morning. Better sleep is the result of a nutrient-rich diet full of organic and whole foods. It's important to understand that whether or not you can have all the hours of sleep you need, this is no guarantee that the quality will be adequate. For example, some people complain about not feeling well-rested, even if they have been in bed for 7-8 hours in total. Chances are, they did not sleep completely during the night, or experienced several interruptions and issues that prevented them from good rest. If you have a lot on your mind, stress or other factors can disrupt good rest, making it difficult to maintain consistent sleep, and avoiding REM (rapid eye movement) or deep sleep.

Stronger Mental Focus and Clarity

A diet high in natural, organic foods without preservatives will improve your brain's health, protecting you against many cognitive diseases and memory loss. Consuming Paleo foods will strengthen your brain's health for decades, including in your mature years.

Healthier Insulin and Blood Glucose Levels

Most Paleo foods are low in carbs, which makes them a better choice for people who are at risk for diabetes and high blood sugar. Carbohydrates are converted into glucose once they are ingested and absorbed, which quickly spikes sugar levels in the body, forcing the pancreas to produce more insulin. This can eventually lead to the development of type 2 diabetes, which can lead to other conditions and medical challenges later in life. By reducing the carbohydrates that you consume, the resistance to insulin is reduced also, which prevents the risk of type 2 diabetes. If you are already diagnosed with diabetes, reducing both your sugar and carb intake will greatly improve your health and prognosis for the future.

Improved Gut Health

Your gut's lining and bacteria will be more balanced, promoting better digestion and microbial balance within your body. Fermented foods are excellent for promoting good digestion, such as kimchi and sauerkraut, both of which are Paleo-friendly and easy to enjoy with a variety of meals, from roast beef, pork chops, chicken or baked salmon, as an example. Sauerkraut is a traditional German dish that is made by fermenting cabbage. Kimchi is a Korean fermented dish that is often spicy and created using cabbage, radishes, or other vegetables. While these fermented foods are great side dishes, they are also ideal as a light meal or snack as well.

Mental Health Benefits

Eating Paleo can reduce the symptoms and effects of depression, anxiety, and related conditions. The natural sugar balance occurs when you avoid processed ingredients, foods, and refined sweeteners and sugars, which can negatively change moods to change erratically and without notice. If you suffer from a mood disorder, you will benefit from Paleo's balanced approach to eating balanced and highly nutritious meals. Studies have indicated the positive effect that nutrient-dense foods have on your cognitive function and the ability to cope with a variety of conditions. While medical treatment may be necessary, eating well will improve the quality of your life and help you achieve a balance.

Increased Energy and Endurance

When you consume natural foods, your body will thrive and reward you with a higher level of energy, as well as endurance. If you plan on joining a marathon or another high-intensity exercise or goal, eating Paleo will take you to the finish line with a sense of renewed energy and satisfaction. By avoiding the high consumption of sugar and foods high in the glycemic index, you can avoid the "crash" that often follows after eating a sweet pastry or another sweetener-filled treat. The amount of natural sugar we need in our diet can be found naturally in fruits and other foods in their whole state, including some vegetables. A sustainable and long-lasting source of energy can be achieved by eating lean sources of protein from lean meats and plant-based foods. As your body utilizes protein sources, muscle tissue is built and strengthened, which lasts far longer than sugar, which is a temporary form of energy, which falls short of any long-term benefits or goals. Endurance is achieved by steadily eating balanced, natural foods as part of the Paleo diet. As you consume more foods high in natural energy, such as fiber, protein, and nutrients, you'll experience a better outcome in all of your physical endeavors and goals.

Reduced Inflammation

Since the Paleo diet has little to not acidic-producing foods, which are often the culprit for inflammation, which is also a side effect of chronic illness and eating foods high in sugar and carbohydrates. The balanced, alkaline-based foods part of the Paleo diet assure that you will not suffer from inflammation due to the low glycemic levels and moderate to high levels of omega 3s, 6s and healthy fats included in this way of eating.

In general, the Paleo diet has plenty of benefits for everyone, and can easily fit into any lifestyle, due to the variety of foods available. It is important to focus on the quality and choice of the foods and ingredients you choose, as opposed to the calories or carbohydrate count, as with many other diets. This type of focus on nutrition means you'll enjoy a higher quality in the meals you consume, along with the reduced sugar, unnatural and refined ingredients, while simply enjoying the foods you choose as a part of your regular eating habits.

BEGINNING THE PALEO DIET

TAKING the First Steps to a Cleaner, Natural Way of Eating

If you're new to the Paleo diet, there are some significant changes to make in the way you eat and choose your food. This can take time and will likely not occur overnight. It's recommended to start slowly by making subtle but meaningful changes that will make a difference over time. Some of the foods we eat may seem harmless, even beneficial if we are led to believe they are good for us. Years ago, campaigns were promoting the consumption of eight glasses of milk each day, without any consideration for allergic reactions and additives that can be found in some types of non-grass fed and processed forms of milk in the grocery stores. Plant-based diets have also received mixed reviews, and while the Paleo diet isn't completely based on vegan eating, it does involve many fresh fruits and vegetables as a significant part of the eating plan. The following two sections detail the most important foods to include in the Paleo diet, as well as the foods that should be avoided at all costs.

Top Foods for the Paleo Diet

There are many foods high in nutritional value that fit within the primal category of the paleo diet and can be included in a variety of meals and snacks. These foods are exemplary for their high nutritional value and provide a good source of nutrients for daily requirements. Consider including options from the following food choices below regularly, to fulfill your nutritional needs.

Dark Green Vegetables

Kale, spinach, and arugula are some of the most nutrient-dense vegetables to include in your daily meal plan to ensure you meet your daily requirements and avoid deficiencies. While all vegetables are highly nutritious, dark greens are strong in iron, calcium, multiple vitamins, and fiber content. As bitter as these vegetables are, they provide a decent base for salads, which can be naturally sweetened with citrus and/or maple syrup and berries. Spinach and arugula provide a good base for salads, or as a way to replace grains, such as rice, beans or pasta, with a serving of chicken, beef or seafood.

Nuts and Seeds

These are an important source of plant-based protein, calcium, and vitamins. Chia seeds contain some of the strongest seeds for nutrient value, with additional vitamins, antioxidants, and other benefits. They are often considered one of the "superfoods" which belong to a group of foods that provide an extremely dense serving of nutrients that can meet the daily requirements for certain vitamins in minerals in just one serving. Almonds, cashews, sesame seeds, sunflower and pumpkin seeds, among many other options, contain an abundance of healthy fats, protein, fiber, vitamins, and calcium. Some Paleo diet follows who prefer a more plant-based approach can find the required daily protein in a daily serving of nuts and/or seeds.

Bananas

A popular snack food, bananas receive special mention because they can provide a significant amount of benefits on their own, or in conjunction with other fruits. Just one banana can provide up to one and a half hours of energy. They not only contain fiber and vitamins but are also a good source of potassium, which helps to prevent inflammation and water retention. Bananas are excellent as a quick snack, and they can also be added to desserts or smoothies to create a tasty treat within a few minutes.

Root Vegetables

Turnips (rutabaga), potatoes, yams, beets, and other root-based vegetables are an excellent source of vitamins, and often provide a natural (unprocessed) form of carbohydrates. These vegetables are not only high in nutrients, but they are also pleasant in flavor and provide a filling side dish or as a main feature in plant-based meals. They are inexpensive and pair well with almost any other ingredients, including any other vegetables, meats, and spices. Carrots and parsnips are also excellent, tasty options to include in your next roast or skillet meal. All varieties of squash, including butternut, acorn, and spaghetti squash, are excellent sources of potassium and beta carotene. Root vegetables also contain a strong source of vitamins, and often enjoyed in a side dish or as part of dinner.

Lean Meats

Red meats such as beef and pork, as well as poultry, can be included in the Paleo diet. A moderate portion of meat is an excellent meal feature with a salad, soup, or baked vegetable. Highly nutritious bone broths, containing collagen, can be created from the bones of a leftover roast or meal. Often, beef and chicken broths are created, though this can be made from fish or other types of meat, including lamb, pork and other cuts of meat. Using meats in a variety of dishes is the best way to enjoy them, and many spices and seasonings can be applied to vary the taste each time. The best way to enjoy meat is to buy in bulk from a local butcher or market and freeze a large portion, using just enough for meals each day.

Seafood

Fish is an excellent source of protein, calcium, and healthy fats. These staple nutrients in a Paleo diet, as they can be found in many primitive food sources from hunting. Any variety of fish is good, and while some

Citrus Fruits

Oranges, lemons, limes, and grapefruit are strong sources of vitamin C and fiber. They tend to be acidic initially, though they become alkaline once ingested. The level of vitamins in these fruits are excellent for the prevention of the common cold and help support and build a stronger immune system. They are also refreshing in taste, whether you enjoy them as they are, include a splash of them in your water or sparkling beverage, or fruit or dark green salad. Grapefruit and oranges are excellent made into freshly squeezed juice, or as an addition to a breakfast meal. They make a wonderful snack during the day. Lemon and lime are often used in homemade dressings and vinaigrette mixes. They are often used in recipes for baking and puddings.

Apples

A strong alkaline food, apples are a good source of energy and vitamin C. They are convenient to enjoy on the go and make an excellent addition to the Paleo diet. Apples are in season in the autumn, when they are best to enjoy, and can be found in many varieties from sour to sweet or a combination in between.

Cabbage, Cauliflower, and Broccoli

Cruciferous vegetables offer a delicious flavor and texture, and can often grow in colder climates, making them easy to find in many regions. They are a good source of fiber, vitamins C, A and K, and iron. They can be enjoyed in a wide variety of dishes, including casseroles, stews, skillet meals, and soups. They are also great for salads in the raw and can be easily shredded and sprinkled over many dishes.

Foods to Avoid on the Paleo Diet

Which foods are best to avoid? For beginners to this diet, it may seem a bit challenging to determine which foods are Paleo-friendly and those that do not fit within this way of eating. Consider the types of foods that were available in primal times, when our ancestors hunted and gathered food, when there was no farming, cultivating, or harvesting done. Like every diet and healthy way of eating, Paleo encourages eating a wide range of whole, natural foods, without the need to count calories or worry about carbohydrates. In following this way of eating, it is imperative to include a wide range of foods that fit within the paleo criteria, while avoiding many other options that will negatively impact your progress. The types of foods that would not be around back then include the following, which are generally not included in the Paleo diet are as follows:

Grains and Legumes

Grains such as oats, wheat, barley, and bran are produced through farming, and for this reason, they are not included in the Paleo diet. Legumes are also farmed or harvested, and not included, as they were not part of the primal diet. Whole grains are a significant part of many meal plans; the Paleo diet easily replaces them with nuts, seeds, greens, and root vegetables.

Bread and Pastries

Bread and pastries are skipped completely on the Paleo diet. This is due to the amount of refined wheat, grains and ingredients used. Pastries are often full of sugar and glazes full of sweeteners and food coloring. Savory pastries may seem like a better option, with fewer sweeteners, though the ingredients include wheat flour that contains a lot of carbohydrates that convert into glucose in the body. Other items in rolls and savory treats may include smoked cheese and meat products, and other processed foods that should be excluded from your diet. If you have a bread craving, some excellent Paleo-friendly recipes include the replacement of wheat, dairy, and sugar ingredients for a better balance in the recipe.

Refined Sugars and Artificial Sweeteners

Any refined or unnatural sugars or sweeteners are completely avoided, and instead, natural sources such as maple syrup, agave, low carb (natural) options, and fruit (which contain fructose) are healthy options for sweetening desserts and drinks. Many pastries and baked goods contain refined sugar and preservatives, which should be avoided, as they can easily spike glucose levels. Artificial sweeteners are often used in place of sugar, which may seem like a good substitute. However, they are full of chemicals and artificial ingredients that can increase other risks to your health. If you want to avoid sugar completely, choose monk fruit or stevia, both of which are natural, sweet and have no impact on increasing blood sugar levels.

Trans Fats and Highly Processed Foods

Deep-fried foods and meals high in trans fats are completely avoided, due to their negative effects on health, and unnatural composition. These foods are responsible for increasing the likelihood of cancer, heart disease, and many other chronic conditions and disorders. Switching French fries for a baked root vegetable or salad is a good option for Paleo, as well as skipping the deep-fried chicken and burgers for a roast, baked, or lightly sautéed version. Onion rings, a popular fast food side, can be reinvented as a baked snack. Zucchini, kale, and pickles can be fried, baked or enjoyed as are in salads or as snacks.

Lot Fat or Zero Fat Foods

Food products labeled as fat-free or having zero fat are not included in the Paleo diet, due to their negative effects on the health. Examples of these foods include packaged cookies, crackers, and dairy products such as flavored yogurt and artisan cheeses. It is best to buy a plain, unsweetened, full-fat version of these foods instead of their artificially sweetened and flavored counterparts, which contain artificial colors, flavors, and hidden sugars. Many "fat-fee" or "low fat" foods are not effective in weight loss either and they are often unable to adequately satisfy hunger.

In general, all foods that are unnatural and include artificial ingredients can be skipped. If in doubt, read labels and choose options from the produce section of the grocery store or farmer's market as often as possible. Skip the grain and legumes aisle completely, and focus on adding root vegetables, in-season fruits, and other vegetables as your main and side features. Meat and dairy are best chosen as organic and with little or no additives. Include as many nuts and seeds as possible, and avoid any varieties with added sugars, coatings or sodium, even if the label promises they are natural. Dried fruits are a good option for a Paleo diet, as long as they are naturally sun-dried instead of chemically dried, which is common. For best options, buy your dried fruits in natural food stores or farmers' markets, where they are from a more natural source or homemade.

The Modified Version of the Paleo Diet

If you are looking for a slight variation from the original Paleo diet, either to gradually follow a full Paleo version or remain with a modified diet, this is a good option. Many people struggle with eliminating certain foods from their diet that are not conducive to Paleo eating. This may be due to having certain allergic restrictions or not being able to access certain foods within their region or immediate area that are Paleo. Easing the restrictions on the Paleo diet is a good way to improve your way of eating, by choosing low glycemic foods and avoiding processed goods, while maintaining decent eating habits. Consider the following criteria for the modified version of the Paleo diet:

- Grass-fed dairy is permitted, and if possible, choose unpasteurized as well. This variety of diary contains no preservatives and is more beneficial for your health as a result. Many farmer's markets, local farms, and some natural food stores may offer this variety of dairy.
- Certain grains and legumes are acceptable to include in a modified Paleo diet, as long as they are soaked, such as beans, to remove some of the additives or phytic acid that are present. By removing these, the beans and other grains become easier to digest. Fermented soybean products, such as miso and tempeh, are good options to include in your diet as well. They are rich in protein, calcium, and B12, and during the fermentation process, the common side effects of soy are removed, which often cause bloating and indigestion for some people. Brown rice, quinoa, buckwheat, and millet are good choices to include, as these grains contain high levels of nutrients. Other grains and

legumes can be enjoyed in moderation, though they should be organic and consumed with other sources of protein, calcium, and fiber.

- Choose gluten-free as much as possible. For example, if you choose to include a small portion of oats in your modified diet, choose gluten-free and organic as much as possible. You may want to include a handful of oats in a bowl of stewed apples with cinnamon, or with a coconut-based yogurt (or grass-fed dairy yogurt).

- Choose coconut oil as much as possible, and include in your daily meals and smoothies, drinks. MCT is the fat extract from coconut oil and can be added as well. The taste is neutral, which makes it an easy addition to many foods and drinks. Other healthy fats to include in your diet include avocado (and avocado oil), olive oil, and sesame oil. Nuts and seeds are also high in good fats and contribute to a balanced diet. These are an important part of the regular Paleo diet and should be included as regularly as possible.

- Root vegetables are a good source of energy and nutrients, though not all varieties are included in the regular Paleo diet, such as potatoes. Sweet potatoes (yams), beets, turnips, and other roots vegetables are good sources of fiber and satisfying in terms of taste and texture. Many of the dishes and recipes you can make with potatoes can be modified to include sweet potato fries or mashed, shredded turnips for hash browns or bakes in the oven, and roasted beets or fries. These types of vegetables allow for a lot of flexibility and options to spice and flavor. You can add them as a side dish or as a main meal. They are great to serve with a steak or serving of roast chicken or salmon.

Modified Paleo embodies the same principles of the regular Paleo,

Maple syrup is another excellent option and a popular choice for pancakes. All of these toppings are paleo-friendly.

- 1 cup of each flour: tapioca and almond (coconut flour can be replaced with half of the almond flour, for a combination of all three, if desired)
- Raw sugar or monk fruit (roughly 2 teaspoons)
- 1 cup of milk (coconut or nut-based milk is recommended; a dairy is also an option)
- Dash of vanilla extract (this ingredient is optional)

With butter or olive oil, heat a skillet to a moderate or medium temperature, and mix the flours and milk with the vanilla extract and sweetener in a bowl, using a whisk to blend thoroughly. Once the batter is smooth, pour 3 or 4-inch diameter portions, one at a time, onto the skillet and cook evenly on both sides, approximately for 2-3 minutes each. Serve with the toppings of your choice.

Spinach and Smoked Salmon Omelet

*I*f you're in the mood for a decadent treat for a weekend brunch or looking to make use of leftover smoked salmon in your refrigerator or freezer, this is an ideal option. Raw or frozen (precooked) spinach can be used in this recipe. If you choose to use fresh spinach, chop it finely after washing and rinsing the leaves thoroughly. Onions and garlic are excellent options to enhance the medley of flavors.

- 3 eggs
- 1 cup of frozen or finely chopped spinach
- ½ cup of diced smoked salmon
- Dash of paprika and black pepper

- Chili powder (optional)
- Fresh dill
- Olive oil for the skillet
- Crushed garlic cloves
- 2 tsp of finely diced or crushed onions

Whisk the eggs, then add in the remaining ingredients, mixing well, then pour onto a heated skillet with olive oil. Cook until the omelet is evenly done, then flip one half over for a minute, followed by flipping the full omelet. Serve garnished or topped with fresh dill or chives.

Mushroom and Ham Omelet

This omelet provides a wealth of protein, calcium, and healthy fats in one meal, and is ideal if you are ready for a busy day at work, or a vigorous exercise at the gym. This dish is low in carbohydrates, which accelerates the metabolism first thing in the morning. If you prefer this type of meal later in the day, it is a great option for lunch or as a light dinner, depending on your schedule. Any variety of mushrooms can be used. Cooked ham sliced into cubes, from a leftover roast, is ideal. If you have leftover roast ham, beef or other red meats in your refrigerator, they can be added to this omelet for a hearty breakfast or brunch.

- 3 eggs
- 1 ½ cups of cooked ham or beef, sliced into cubes or small pieces
- Black pepper and sea salt
- Dill, dried or fresh
- Fresh chives or grated onion, about 2 tablespoons
- Paprika, about 1 teaspoon

- Dash of chili pepper (optional)
- Olive oil
- Thinly sliced mushrooms, about ½ cup

Whisk the three eggs into a bowl, then add in the mushrooms, cubed meat, seasoning, and spices, including onion or chives, and other spices as desired. Heat a skillet with the olive oil, and gently pour in the egg mix to cook evenly for about 2-3 minutes. When the one side is cooked, lift half and fold over to the other, then gently flip and cook for another 2-3 minutes or until well done. Serve with a slice of Paleo bread, fresh greens or fruit salad.

Fruit Salad for Breakfast

*W*hether you enjoy a full breakfast with fruit on the side, or a simple bowl of fruit to get started, this is an ideal option to consider in the morning, or as a mid-morning snack. The fruits you choose for this salad are plenty, though it is best to pick foods in season, as they are fresh and easy to find at local markets. There are many fruits available year-round as well, whether fresh or frozen, including berries, mangoes, bananas, apples, and kiwi. If you decide to include fruits only available frozen, allow them to defrost at least one hour before adding to the recipe. If you pick apples for your fruit salad, add a little lemon juice to them to prevent them from turning brown, which can happen quickly.

- 1 ½ - 2 cups of fresh berries (blackberries, strawberries, blueberries, currants and/or raspberries)
- 1 sliced banana
- 2 kiwis, sliced
- 1 cup of sliced mango or pineapple chunks

- Sliced apple (1 small or medium)
- Orange or mandarin pieces (8-10)
- Fresh lemon juice

Combine the above ingredients into a large bowl and sprinkle lemon juice, freshly squeezed, over the fruits. Serve as a side with poached or fried eggs, or with a dollop of grass-fed yogurt.

Fried Eggs With Bacon and Spinach

*A*traditional breakfast, eggs, and bacon can be enjoyed as a weekend brunch or during the week. The best way to prepare bacon and minimize fried oils and grease is to bake them in the oven before preparing the eggs and spinach. Frozen spinach is a convenient option, as it is already cooked, and compressed into serving sizes. The equivalent of ½ cup of spinach is usually one serving in a frozen package of spinach. Alternatively, if you use fresh spinach, this can be served as a side with a light vinaigrette dressing.

- 1 cup of fresh or ½ cup of cooked spinach
- 3 eggs
- 4 slices of bacon
- Olive oil
- Sea salt and black pepper
- Paprika

Set the bacon in the oven on a baking tray, lightly greased with olive oil. Bake for 8-10 minutes, then monitor until crispy, at 350 degrees, then remove to cool. Prepare the eggs on a skillet with olive oil, and fry over-easy. Toss in the spinach, if cooked, or if raw, toss in a bowl with lemon vinaigrette. Serve the eggs over the spinach with the bacon on the side. Sprinkle sea salt, black pepper, and paprika on top. Serve over the spinach (raw or cooked) and add the bacon. If desired, crumble the bacon and sprinkle over the eggs. Paleo bread can be served with this meal, or a sliced grapefruit or orange.

Egg Breakfast Bites

*I*f you are looking for a breakfast-to-go option that can be prepared the night before, consider making these small, bite-sized breakfast treats that can be easily microwaved or reheated to go in the morning. All you need is a muffin tray, silicone or paper cups, and a few ingredients:

- 6 eggs, large (or 7-8 medium or small eggs)
- ½ cup of shredded sharp cheddar (unpasteurized and grass-fed)
- 2 tablespoons of crumbled crispy bacon or bacon bits
- 1 tablespoon of chives, finely chopped
- Sea salt and black pepper
- Paprika
- Chili pepper (or crushed dried chilies)

Whisk all the eggs in a large bowl, and toss in the paprika, sea salt, and black pepper. Add in the chives, chili pepper (optional), crispy bacon and shredded cheddar, and combine until all ingredients are evenly mixed. Pour into 6 silicone or paper muffin cups lining a tray, then place it in a preheated oven. Bake for approximately 12-14 minutes or until the egg cups are well done, then remove from the oven and serve after cooling for a few minutes. These breakfast bites can be refrigerated and enjoyed up to 3 days or added to the freezer for up to one month. Several batches can be prepared at once by doubling or tripling the recipe contents. Other ingredients to consider for this recipe:

- Cubed or shredded pieces of cooked ham
- Sliced and sautéed mushrooms (cook first, then add to egg cups)
- Lightly sautéed garlic or garlic powder
- Fresh parsley or dill, shredded, or dried

Lunch and Light Meals

Whether you enjoy a mid-morning snack in between breakfast and lunch or skip right to the middle meal of the day, it's important to include a good source of nutrients to boost your energy levels, which may be spent since the morning. Since rice, pasta, and grains are not used as a base for Paleo dishes, root vegetables, dark greens, and sprouts are often a good choice. Like low carb and ketogenic diets, paleo dishes may include "riced" or finely grated cauliflower or broccoli in place of rice, or spiral yams or zucchini instead of wheat pasta.

Beef or Poultry Bone Broth

*R*ecently, the health benefits of collagen and nutrient contained in beef and poultry bones have become popularly enjoyed as a broth. While common beef, chicken and vegetable broths are available in stores, a bone broth requires deep saturation of bones stewed in boiling water for at least 20-24 hours. The best way to obtain bones for preparing your home-made broth is by visiting your local butcher for leftover bones from cuts of meat, or the remainder of roast beef, turkey or chicken dinner. Other meat bones such as pork and venison can be used, though poultry and beef are the most common and popular in the Paleo diet. To prepare, add the bones of one carcass to 6-8 cups of water and boil until bubbling. Continue to boil for at least half an hour, then reduce and stew for another hour on moderately low. After this point, you can continue stewing the bones on low heat, adding your desired medley of spices, including sea salt, black pepper, savory, thyme, sage, chili powder, etc. Cover and stew on low for several hours. If you need to leave the area, turn the stove off completely and cover it until the next day. Remove from the stove after a total of 20-24 hours and use it as desired.

Ingredients for bone broth:

- Bones of one carcass or meal (1 chicken, turkey or roast beef)
- Sea salt
- Black pepper
- Desired spices and seasoning: chili pepper, thyme, oregano, savory, etc.

Bone broth can be stored in the refrigerator in a jar or resealable container for up to one week, or the freezer for up to 3 months.

Skillet Cauliflower and Bacon Crumble

An aromatic and delicious vegetable, cauliflower is a mild, yet textured and tasty vegetable that combines well with many ingredients and flavors. This dish is easy to prepare and includes the addition of crumbled, crispy bacon that is best to prepare first or kept from breakfast or lunch leftovers. If you plan on making this dish and decide to include bacon with your breakfast, fry some extra to prepare for this meal in advance.

- 1 head of cauliflower, sliced into small florets, about 2-3 cups
- Butter, unsalted, for the skillet (olive oil can also be used)
- ½ or ¾ cups of bacon crumble
- Parmesan cheese, grated or dried
- Crushed garlic cloves, about 2 (finely diced or garlic powder)
- Sea salt and black better
- Paprika

Melt the butter in the skillet with the garlic, sea salt, pepper, and paprika. Saute for 2-3 minutes on moderate heat, before tossing in the cauliflower florets. Continue to cook, coating the cauliflower florets, sautéing them continuously until they are coated and lightly golden. Add in the parmesan cheese, approximately 2-3 teaspoons, and more butter, if needed. When the cauliflower is nearly done, fold in the bacon crumble and continue to stir lightly for a few minutes, then serve. Top with additional parmesan and/or parsley, if desired.

Skillet Portobello Mushrooms With Onions

*P*ortobello mushrooms are a nutrient-rich food that can be enjoyed as a main meal feature with onions, spices and other vegetables that can be tasty in a skillet. This dish is easy to create, using olive or avocado oil with fresh portobello mushroom caps.

- Portobello mushroom caps, 4 in total
- Olive oil
- Sea salt and black pepper
- Chili powder or dried chilies

- Paprika
- Sliced onion, 1 medium or large

Place the portobello mushroom caps in a heated skillet with olive or avocado oil and saute for a few minutes on each side. Toss in the onion slices, and saute once the mushrooms are nearly done, cooking them together. Top with the seasoning and spices, then serve with salad or as a light meal.

Lettuce and Tuna Wraps

*B*read and whole wheat wraps are not included in the Paleo diet, though lettuce wraps can substitute well, and provide a good option for holding a lot of ingredients and toppings. Canned tuna is convenient and best to use for this meal, though baked tuna is another option, especially if it is leftover from a previous dinner. Combine tuna with the following ingredients and add into a large lettuce leaf:

- 1 can of tuna, drained (water-based, not oil)
- Olive oil
- Chopped onion, about 2 tablespoons
- Chili powder
- Sea salt and black pepper

Drain the tuna from the can, and mash into a bowl with the olive oil, onion, and chili powder. Add in the sea salt and black pepper, and some of the following ingredients, as desired:

- Dried parsley or dill
- Chives, fresh or dried
- Mashed avocado

- Dash of lime or lemon juice

Scoop the mixture onto the lettuce leaf, then wrap and enjoy. This recipe will make approximately two leaf wraps.

Cucumber, Tuna and Arugula Salad

*L*ike tuna salad wraps, this recipe uses the same recipe as above and combines it with chunkier cuts of vegetables for a salad dish. This can be easily enjoyed as a full lunch on its own, or with soup. This salad contains major ingredients that are required in everyday meals, including protein, fiber, calcium, and vitamins. While the recipe includes cucumbers and arugula, there are many other ingredient possibilities available to change the flavor of this dish.

- Can of tuna, drained
- 1 small shallot, diced
- ½ cucumber (large) or a small cucumber, sliced into small ½-inch pieces
- 1 cup of arugula, diced
- Sea salt and black pepper
- Chili pepper (optional)
- Olive oil
- Lemon juice
- Dill or parsley (or both), dried or freshly chopped

Combine all the ingredients in a bowl, beginning with the tuna, mixing with the olive oil, sea salt, black pepper, lemon juice, chili pepper, and dill or parsley. Add in the cucumber and arugula, once the other ingredients are well combined, then serve.

Paleo Bread

. . .

*S*ince grains and baked goods are avoided on the Paleo diet, it can be challenging to find the alternative. This bread recipe is perfect for Paleo, as it contains only the diet-friendly ingredients, avoiding all grains and dairy. This is a loaf that can be created in your oven at home for any occasion and creates an excellent style of bread for any sandwich you choose to make.

- Almond Flour, 2 cups
- Coconut Flour, 2 tablespoons
- Baking soda, about 1 teaspoon
- Flaxseed meal or ground flax seeds, about ½ cups
- Arrowroot or tapioca flour, about ½ cup
- Baking powder, about 1 tablespoon
- Dash of sea salt
- 1/8 cups of almond or cashew milk
- 2 egg whites
- 3 large eggs
- 1 teaspoon of apple cider vinegar
- Coconut oil, about ¼ cups

Mix all the dry ingredients listed above in a large bowl, then set aside. Whisk the egg whites (2) in one bowl, and separately, the whole eggs (3) in another bowl. Stir in the dry mixture with the wet, and add in the almond or cashew milk, apple cider vinegar, coconut oil and eggs (egg whites and whole eggs). Move all the batter to a prepared baking loaf and set inside a preheated oven. Bake for 30 minutes or until loaf is done. This bread can be stored up to one week in the refrigerator.

Dinner Recipes

The final meal of the day doesn't have to be elaborate or time-consuming to be healthy and reasonable. Dinners can be a simple feast for one or two or a combination of several dishes and options for a family or larger household or group of people. The options in this section include both features of the main meal and the sides. These can be mixed and matched depending on your preference, and whether you prefer to include meat as a feature or more plant-based options. Many foods, both meat-based, and vegetables, can be prepared easily in the oven or skillet.

Baked Salmon With Dill and Parsley

*J*f you're a fan of salmon, one of the healthiest fish options to include in your diet, this dish is easy to prepare in the oven as you create side dishes. Frozen or fresh salmon steaks are ideal for this recipe, which are simply baked in a dish for 45 minutes with lemon juice and seasoning, and served with fresh lemon, dill, and parsley.

- Lemon juice (for coating the salmon steaks)
- 3-4 salmon steaks
- Black pepper, sea salt, fresh or dried dill
- Fresh parsley
- Olive oil (or avocado oil)
- Paprika and thyme

Coat the salmon steaks lightly in lemon juice, and place in a baking dish or tray lightly greased with olive oil or avocado oil. Coat lightly in seasoning (black pepper, sea salt, thyme, and paprika) and bake in the oven for 45-50 minutes at 350 degrees. Check periodically and remove once the fish is flaky and well done. Serve with additional fresh squeezed lemon juice, and garnish with dill and parsley. Serve with fresh arugula or spinach and/or ripe avocado as aside. A roasted root vegetable is another excellent option to serve with salmon.

Chicken Kale and Garlic Skillet

*T*his is an easy and quick skillet dish to make with chicken breast, garlic, kale and sesame oil with your choice of seasoning and spices. In this recipe, dried chilies, garlic powder, and cumin are recommended. For a savory taste, without heat, try combining savory, sage, thyme, and oregano combined. Chicken is versatile and provides an excellent source of lean protein. Sesame seeds are a great option as a topping for this dish, either raw or toasted.

- 1 pound of boneless, skinless chicken breast (organic is recommended)
- 3 cups of finely diced or shredded kale, with stems, removed
- Crushed garlic (grated or crushed, about 3 cloves)
- Sesame oil for frying
- Dried chilies or powder
- Black pepper and sea salt
- Dry roasted or raw sesame seeds
- Additional seasoning/spices to consider savory, thyme, oregano, etc.

Cut the boneless chicken into one-inch pieces, or slightly larger, and add to a skillet with sesame oil. Cook at a moderate temperature for 5-6 minutes, then toss in the garlic and spices. Continue to saute until chicken is well done, then reduce heat to low and toss in shredded kale. In another skillet, lightly toast the sesame seeds on moderate to high heat for 1-2 minutes, then set aside (raw sesame seeds can be used without toasting). Serve the sauteed chicken, garlic, and kale with spices sprinkled with sesame seeds on top.

Roasted Yams

*a*n excellent side dish, or as the main feature of a plant-based meal. Yams or sweet potatoes are excellent sources of vitamin A and fiber and can be easily prepared in the oven, much like regular potatoes. To prepare yams, scrub and wash them vigorously, then slice them in 3 or 4-inch pieces and add to a roasting pan. They usually take anywhere between 45-60 minutes to roast fully, and this timeframe should be taken into consideration when preparing other dishes or sides to serve together so that they are all done at the same time. Roasting yams in a medium pan or baking dish include the following simple ingredients:

- 3-4 yams or sweet potatoes (sliced into smaller pieces, about 3 or 4-inches in size)
- Paprika, thyme, sea salt, and black pepper
- Olive oil or butter
- Fresh parsley
- Sour cream (full fat, unsweetened). Plain Greek or Icelandic yogurt can also be used in place of sour cream

Prepare the baking tray or dish by coating with a thin layer of butter or olive oil, and place the yams inside, lightly sprinkling with olive oil or butter, sea salt, and the remaining spices. If some heat is desired, add a dash of cayenne, chili pepper, and/or Cajun spice. Bake, covered, in the oven for approximately 45-60 minutes, checking every 30 minutes on the progress. Depending on the oven and the size of the potatoes, the baking may take more or less time. Once the yams are tender, remove from the oven and serve topped with fresh butter (at room temperature), a dollop of sour cream and a dash of paprika on top with fresh parsley.

Broccoli, Cheese and Bacon Crumble Bake

 $\mathcal{T}$ his is a delicious casserole that combines the delicious taste of baked broccoli and a variety of cheeses of your preference of unpasteurized, grass-fed cheese. While the Paleo diet doesn't typically include diary, unpasteurized dairy can be an option. This recipe includes shredding and mixing any 3-4 varieties of cheese to mix and top with the broccoli. This provides an in-depth medley of cheese taste, which complements the vegetables well.

- 1 head of broccoli, sliced into small florets
- 3-4 cups of shredded cheese, any type, and varieties. (Sharp or old cheddar is recommended, along with mozzarella, gouda and/or Monterey Jack or Swiss cheese).
- Butter at room temperature or olive oil
- Sea salt, black pepper, and paprika
- Almond flour and parmesan cheese (for the topping)

Toss the broccoli floret pieces with the shredded cheese, mixing evenly, then pour into a lightly greased casserole dish (with butter or olive oil). Ensure the cheese and broccoli are combined evenly, so there are no areas with little or no cheese. Mix the sea salt, black pepper, and paprika in a bowl with the parmesan cheese and almond flour (about 1-2 teaspoons each for the almond flour and parmesan cheese), then sprinkle carefully and evenly over the top of the casserole, before placing in the oven. Bake at 350 degrees for approximately 35-45 minutes, until the top is a light golden or brown color, then remove to slice and serve.

If you don't have enough broccoli or would like to mix the vegetable with other options, consider creating in the same casserole with the addition of sliced carrots, cauliflower florets, and/or parsnips.

Paleo Chili

*T*raditionally, chili is made with beans and legumes, which is where this recipe differs significantly. Vegetables such as zucchini, celery, carrots, onions, and dark greens take the place of beans. Tomatoes and garlic, along with chili powder and spices remain in this dish, along with lean ground beef. If you want an interesting twist on this dish, consider switching the beef with lamb or pork, or combining two different types of meats. Alternatively, this chili can be created as a vegan dish by skipping meat completely.

- Lean ground beef, about 1 pound
- 2 teaspoons of chili powder
- Sea salt and black pepper
- Crushed or pureed tomatoes, about 4 cups
- Onion, about 1/2 cup diced
- Crushed garlic cloves or powder
- Celery, chopped, about 1 cup
- Zucchini, small or medium, diced
- Carrots, diced
- Mushrooms, sliced thinly
- Olive oil for sauteing the beef

*A*dd the beef or lean ground meat of your choice to a heated skillet with olive oil, and cook well until brown, then add the onions, garlic, spices, and saute for a few more minutes, at a moderate temperature. Add all the vegetables and continue to cook. Saute until the vegetables are tender, then add the contents of the skillet to a large cooking pot to begin stewing the chili. Cook on low or a slightly moderate to low temperature, stirring in the tomato sauce, additional spices and if desired, more tomato sauce or diced tomatoes. Serve in a bowl as a main dish or light lunch.

Chicken Breast Skillet Meal With Greens

*T*his is a delicious meal with slices of chicken breast marinated with sesame seed oil and spices, cooked with a handful of spinach and kale, or an assortment of greens, including broccoli, arugula and/or cabbage. This skillet meal is highly nutritious and ideal for a boost of energy for later in the day. Ideally, if there is enough food left, you can set aside a portion or two for leftovers the next day. If desired, set aside for up to 3-4 days in the refrigerator. Skillet meals with meat tend to marinate more after at least one day, allowing the various flavors included to saturate and strengthen the taste.

- 2 chicken breast, boneless, cut into smaller, bite-sized pieces
- Sesame oil, to marinate the chicken
- Olive oil, for the skillet
- 1 cup of raw spinach

- Arugula, (approx. ½ cup), raw
- 1 cup of diced broccoli florets
- 1 cup of shredded cabbage
- 1-2 cups of other vegetables, as desired
- Sesame seeds, about 1 tablespoon
- 2 teaspoons of orange juice and zest
- Crushed garlic cloves, about 1-2
- Shredded or grated onion, about ¼ cup

*N*ote: it is ideal to marinate the chicken in sesame oil and orange juice overnight, to strengthen the taste before adding to the skillet.

*T*he skillet is prepared by adding the olive oil and placing the chicken pieces inside. After a few minutes, add in the onion, garlic, and seasoning, sautéing for another 8-10 minutes, until the chicken is tender, and the spices and ingredients added so far are saturated into the chicken. If there is any sesame oil or orange zest or juice are leftover from marinating, or no margination is done before this dish, add into the skillet as the chicken is cooking with the spices. After a few minutes, add in the remaining ingredients and simmer at a moderate temperature until all the ingredients are tender. Serve sprinkled with sesame seeds.

Cashew Beef, Asparagus, and Chili Peppers

*S*tewing beef is ideal for this recipe, or a similar cut of beef sliced into one or two-inch pieces. Cashews offer an excellent layer of texture and taste to a sautéed dish of beef with asparagus and olive oil. Chili pepper is used to spice the plate as the beef is cooked. The asparagus takes a while to cook and can either be steamed before adding to the skillet, or adding in sooner, as the beef is cooking.

- 1 pound of beef, sliced into cubes
- 1 cup of coarsely chopped cashews, or whole (these can be dry roasted)
- Chili peppers, dried or in powder form
- ½ bunch of asparagus, sliced in half
- Olive oil
- Crushed garlic cloves

Toss the cubed beef into a prepared skillet with olive oil and saute for a few minutes, then add in the garlic, chili pepper, and asparagus. The beef will take a while to cook, as will the asparagus, which can either be sautéed in the same skillet or separately. Cook for at least 15-18 minutes, then serve with lightly dry roasted cashews as a topping.

Lamb Burgers

These are a tasty meal option that can be enjoyed with any variety of fresh toppings, including caramelized onions and greens. Ground lamb is the ideal option, though beef or chicken are also options (these recipes can be found below).

. . .

Ground lamb, 1 pound

Almond flour, 1/2 cup

1 egg

Tarragon, 1 teaspoon

Sea salt and black pepper

Dill or parsley, dried or fresh and diced

Olive oil

Use the olive oil to heat the skillet to a moderate temperature, while preparing the ingredients in a bowl. Combine the ground lamb, egg, sea salt, black pepper, parsley, and tarragon. Mix well until all ingredients are evenly distributed, then form burger patties and fry individually on the skillet, about 3-5 minutes on each side. Serve on a lettuce leaf or as is, with some of the following toppings:

Guacamole, freshly made, or sliced avocado

Sliced tomatoes

Fresh or caramelized onions

Fresh spinach or arugula

Pesto

Fresh dill or parsley

Mustard

Black olives, pitted and sliced

Jalapeno pepper

Chicken Meatballs

*T*his dish is baked in the oven with tomato sauce and a combination of spices and seasoning. Beef or pork can be substituted when chicken is unavailable.

*G*round chicken, lean, about 1 pound

1 teaspoon of garlic powder

Sea salt and black pepper

Olive oil

Savory spice

Paprika

Thyme

1 egg

1/4 cup of almond flour

*I*n a large bowl, combine the ground chicken with the egg, sea salt, black pepper, and seasoning. Mix well, then add in the almond flour, combining evenly. Form the mixture into 1-inch balls or one and a half-inch in diameter, then place on a prepared baking sheet. Bake in the oven at 350 degrees for 35-45 minutes, until done, then serve with your choice of tomato sauce.

Garlic Shrimp With Spinach and Lemon

*T*his is an ideal dinner option if you have shrimp in the freezer. This is a simple meal that doesn't require a lot of preparation and can be prepared in a matter of minutes. Spinach tends to shrink when it is cooked, and for this reason, two cups or one bunch of spinach is good for a sizable serving. One pound of shrimp is ideal, and in large size, though a slightly larger or smaller serving will work for this recipe. The feature of this meal is the garlic and spices used to enhance the experience.

- 1 pound of shrimp (large, jumbo shrimp) or medium in size
- Crushed cloves of garlic (about 2-3)
- Dill, dried or fresh
- Olive oil
- Sea salt and black pepper
- 2 cups of raw spinach, washed and trimmed
- Sliced mushrooms (optional)

Olive oil is used to heat the skillet to medium, then add in the shrimp. If cooking from frozen, allow enough time to cook thoroughly, about 8-10 minutes, then add in the garlic, black pepper, sea salt, and dill. Add in the spinach and cook on moderate, ensuring all the leaves are fully cooked, and begin to shrink. Toss in the mushrooms, when the shrimp and spinach are almost done, then cook for a couple of more minutes, before removing to serve with sliced lemon.

Other options to consider for this recipe include:

- Adding roasted or raw almonds to the stir fry or skillet, when preparing this meal
- A dash of crushed chili peppers
- Fresh paprika, sprinkled on the dish to serve
- Leftover, cooked chicken breast from a roast or previous stir fry

Meal Replacements and Smoothies

Life is busy for most people, which makes preparing a full meal often challenging. If you encounter busy mornings or hectic schedules that don't allow for much meal planning, having a selection of snacks and go-to items to grab on your commute or errands.

Avocado and Coconut Milk Smoothie

*C*oconut and avocadoes contain a wealth of healthy fats, along with a good source of nutrients, including vitamins and fiber. This Smoothie combines the pleasant flavors of avocado and coconut with maple syrup or a low carb sweetener for a satisfying replacement for a quick drink.

- Coconut milk (1 cup)
- Avocado (ripened, soft)
- Maple syrup (1-2 tbsp)
- Coconut cream (optional)

Mix all the ingredients in a blender and pulse until the result is smooth. Serve immediately. As an option, add a banana with another cup of milk.

Mango and Kefir Smoothie

. . .

*M*angoes are a good source of vitamin A, C, and fiber. Combining them with kefir, a stronger fermented yogurt drink, is an ideal way to strengthen gut health and microbial balance in the body. Kefir can be found in grocery stores and natural food markets. It's best to choose plain, unsweetened and unflavored kefir, instead of the flavored options, which often include hidden sugars and artificial flavors.

- Mangoes (1 large or 2 small)
- 1 cup of kefir
- Coconut or almond milk (1 cup)
- Maple syrup or raw sugar

Mix the ingredients and blend for 40 seconds, then taste test and add more milk and/ or sweetener as needed. Continue to blend, then serve.

Peanut Butter and Chocolate Smoothie

*T*his smoothie combines the sweetness of chocolate with the protein and calcium richness of peanut butter. Cashew, almond or another nut butter can be used in place of peanut butter if desired. Smooth nut-butter is the best option without added sugar or sodium. The smooth texture mixes well with the cocoa or chocolate and blends easier in the food processor or blender.

- Coconut or almond milk (2 cups)
- Smooth, unsalted and sugar-free peanut butter (1 cup)
- ½ cup of melted chocolate or the equivalent in dark cocoa powder, unsweetened

- Maple syrup (1-2 tbsp)
- Coconut cream (optional)
- Dash of vanilla or almond extract

Mash the peanut butter and melted chocolate or cocoa powder together, then add in the sweetener, coconut cream, and vanilla or almond extract. Scoop into a blender and add in the two cups of coconut or almond milk, then pulse for 45-60 seconds, until smooth, then serve.

Banana and Pistachio Smoothie

*B*ananas are a powerful form of energy, providing a significant dose of fiber and potassium to any dish they are added. In a smoothie, their nutritional value is strong, as they are raw and enjoyed immediately. Pistachios are a tasty, green nut that pairs well with the taste of bananas, providing additional protein, healthy fats, and calcium.

- 1 ripe banana
- ¼ cup of shelled, raw pistachios (without sodium or sugar)
- Dash of sea salt
- 2 cups of almond, dairy or coconut milk
- Dash of vanilla extract
- Maple syrup, agave or a low carb sweetener

Mash the ripe banana in a bowl with the vanilla extract, sweetener, and sea salt. In a grinder, blend the raw, shelled pistachios until they resemble a fine powder. Add into the bowl and mix, then scoop into a blender or food processor with the milk, and pulse for about 45-60 minutes, until smooth. Serve topped with a sprinkle of cardamom or cinnamon.

Almond Butter and Cocoa Cups

$\mathcal{T}$he combination of almond and cocoa is not only delicious but healthy and full of nutrients. Dark chocolate contains antioxidants, while almond butter is a good source of protein, healthy fats, and calcium. These cups are prepared without the use of baking, and only require a small saucepan to melt the chocolate which can be done with coconut oil or grass-fed butter.

- ½ cup of smooth almond butter, preferably organic
- 6-8 squares of dark chocolate (baker's chocolate)
- 2 teaspoons of agave or maple syrup (low carb sweetener can also be used)
- 1 teaspoon of coconut oil or softened butter

To prepare for this recipe, add silicone or paper cups to a muffin tray. These cups contain three layers: chocolate on the top and bottom and almond butter in the center. The baker's chocolate is melted in a small saucepan on medium with coconut oil and sweetener at a low temperature to prevent burning. When the chocolate is completely melted, remove from the stove and cool for a few minutes. Gently scoop enough chocolate to fill ¼ or ½ inches at the bottom of each cup. Depending on the size of the cups, this may fill 6-8 muffin cups and should leave enough for the top layer. Place in the freezer for 15-20 minutes, which will allow the chocolate to harden. Remove after this time frame and scoop enough almond butter to fill about ½ inch for the second layer or center of each cup.

Return the muffin tray to the freezer for another 15-20 minutes, or until the almond butter has hardened. Remove to add the final layer of chocolate on top and return to the freezer for the final 15-

20 minutes. After the final set, the cups are immediately ready to serve. They can also be left in the freezer for longer, or transferred to the refrigerator, though should onlu6be removed when ready to enjoy, as they will quickly melt at room temperature. These snacks are also referred to as ketogenic or keto "fat bombs," as they contain a good portion of healthy fats and energy, with moderate protein. The keto version includes low carb sweetener, though, in Paleo, any natural, unrefined sugar or sweetener can be added.

Coconut Blueberry Cheesecake Cups

*T*his is a delicious treat that can be easily created using the same muffin tray arrangement like the above recipe. These cups provide the rich, satisfying taste of cheesecake without the sugars or artificial flavors. Full-fat, unsweetened or unflavored cream cheese is used for this recipe, including the addition of plain, shredded coconut and frozen or fresh blueberries.

- 2 cups of plain, unsweetened and unflavored cream cheese
- Fresh or frozen blueberries
- 2-3 tablespoons of shredded coconut (unsweetened)
- Pinch of vanilla extract
- 2-3 teaspoons of maple syrup, agave or low carb sweetener

Before using the cream cheese, ensure it is softened at room temperature. If using from the refrigerator, microwave for approximately 30-40 seconds, until it is softened, and easy to mix with other ingredients. Mash the cream cheese, shredded coconut, sweetener, and sweetener, and combine well, so there are no uneven chunks of ingredients, and none of the items are clumped together. Gently fold in the blueberries, and scoop into silicone or paper muffin cups, filling approximately 2/3 or ¾ full each. Set in the freezer for about 20-25 minutes, then serve. These treats are full of protein and fiber and make an excellent snack before the gym or in the summer during a quick dash outside to work or errands. Keep these cups in the refrigerator or freezer until serving, as they will melt at room temperature.

Coconut and Pineapple Smoothie

A tropical-themed recipe, this smoothie is refreshing and ideal during the summer months.

2 cups of coconut milk

1 cup of pineapple chunks, fresh or frozen

Raw sugar or maple syrup

Vanilla collagen protein powder (optional), 1 tablespoon

I n a blender, combine the ingredients and pulse for at least 40 seconds. Add more of the ingredients, if needed, or ice to this drink to cool down if the pineapple isn't frozen. Papaya or mango can be added as well, or used in place of the pineapple

Cocoa and Cashew Nut Smoothie

A rich-tasting smoothie and without dairy, this smoothie is a decadent combination of cashew milk, butter, and cocoa powder.

. . .

2 cups of cashew milk

Cocoa powder, about 2 tablespoons

Raw sugar or maple syrup

Cocoa or vanilla collagen powder (optional), 1 tablespoon

1 ripe banana, optional

*C*ombine all the ingredients and blend for 35-45 seconds, then serve.

Desserts

Sweets and treats can be enjoyed as part of a balanced Paleo diet, which includes a wide range of natural ingredients, including fruits, unrefined sweeteners, milk, cream, nuts, and seeds. These recipes are simple and tasty, without all the artificial and refined ingredients often found in the baked goods, pastries, puddings, and custards.

Vanilla and Raspberry Chia Seed Pudding

*T*his is a simple recipe to create with a few ingredients. Chia seeds are a rich source of many nutrients, including antioxidants, calcium, protein, and fiber. There are many variations of chia seed pudding recipes, including this basic vanilla flavor, with the addition of frozen or fresh raspberries. Chia seed puddings are best prepared the night before, as they "gel" with milk or yogurt overnight in the refrigerator, ready for enjoyment the following day.

- ¾ cups of chia seeds
- ½ cup of fresh or frozen raspberries
- Maple syrup or low carb sweetener
- 2 cups of milk (dairy or nut-based milk; coconut milk is another option)
- Dash of vanilla extract
- 2 teaspoons of cream, either dairy or coconut cream

Pour the milk and cream into a bowl and whisk together, while adding in the sweetener, vanilla extract, and chia seeds. Ensure all the ingredients are well combined before stirring in the raspberries. Refrigerate overnight, or for a minimum of two hours, then enjoy.

Chocolate Chia Pudding

*L*ike the recipe above, this tasty dish includes the infusion of rich, dark chocolate, which can be melted in advance or used in cocoa powder form, combined with coconut oil and natural sweetener. To melt chocolate, unsweetened baker's chocolate is the best option or another bar chocolate that is roughly 85-90% or more in cocoa content. The higher the percentage of cocoa, the more nutrient-dense the result, and less sugar.

- ¾ cups of chia seeds
- ½ bar of dark chocolate (baker's chocolate or cocoa powder)
- Maple syrup or low carb sweetener
- 2 cups of milk (coconut or nut-based milk; coconut milk is another option). Chocolate almond or nut-based milk is an option, though it's important to check if there are artificial sugars or flavors before including.

- 1-2 teaspoons of cocoa powder
- 2 teaspoons of cream, either dairy or coconut cream

Melt the baker's chocolate slowly on a low temperature in a saucepan with coconut oil and sweetener until the result is smooth without any lumps or clumps. Once this is achieved, remove from the stove, or keep on the burner and shut off the stove. Cool for a few minutes before adding to the coconut milk, cream, whisking thoroughly, then adding in the cocoa powder, chia seeds, and additional sweetener, if desired. Taste test to ensure the sweetness level is to your liking, and ensure the chia seeds are well mixed, then refrigerate overnight or for a couple of hours, then enjoy. When serving, top with dark chocolate chips or shavings.

Paleo Brownies

*I*t is possible to create a delicious baked recipe without processed wheat or grains. This recipe replaces whole wheat with tapioca flour and almond flour. Coconut oil is also used, along with coconut sugar, both of which are Paleo-friendly. These brownies are easy to prepare and bake in the oven within half an hour.

- Coconut oil, about ½ cup
- Dark chocolate chips, about 1 cup (chocolate shavings will also work)
- 3 tablespoons of cocoa powder
- Tapioca flour, about ½ cup
- Sea salt
- 3 eggs
- Vanilla extract

- Espresso powder (optional) or crushed coffee beans, about 1 teaspoon
- Almond flour or crushed almonds, 1 tablespoon

Melt the chocolate chips and coconut oil in a saucepan on low heat or in a microwave for 20 seconds. In a mixing bowl, add the coconut sugar, flours, eggs, sea salt, and espresso powder. Combine well, then blend with an electric or manual hand-held mixer for about one minute. Fold in the melted chocolate with coconut oil and use the mixer to combine evenly. Pour the batter into a prepared baking loaf pan and set inside a preheated oven to bake at 350 degrees for 25-30 minutes. Use a toothpick to determine when the brownies are done. Remove from the oven to cool for a few minutes, then slice and serve. Sprinkle flakes of sea salt on each brownie, if desired.

LIFESTYLE AND THE PALEO DIET

The Importance of Exercise

Staying active and getting enough exercise is one of the most important ways you can stay healthy with a balanced diet. This does not require athletic feats of movement or becoming a daily gym guest, though the more you work out, the better you will utilize the nutrients in a Paleo diet and use them to benefit your body overall.

Finding the Right Exercise and Dietary Routine for Long-term Results and Lifetime Benefits

Exercise and working out means something different to everyone. If you walk once a day for an hour, this may be enough for your ability and fitness level, whereas other people may engage in high impact sports or more strenuous exercise to achieve certain results. Different types of movement and activities that are important for a balanced lifestyle include the following:

- Yoga, stretching, and mindful mediation. This is a great way to relieve stress, realign your focus and increase your flexibility.
- Weight training and lifting are essential ways to build muscle and tone
- Aerobics and cardiovascular exercise are important for weight loss and overall toning. It's a great way to increase endurance and your fitness level
- Cycling, swimming, jogging, sprinting, and team sports are all examples of how to stay in shape. Also, dance lessons, martial arts, and tai chi are excellent options as well.

Bonus Recipes for On the Go

Do you need a quick snack or serving of nutrients and energy on the go? These recipes are ideal for making something in a pinch.

Crispy Kale Chips

*I*f you're looking for a healthy snack that can be prepared in a matter of minutes, this is an ideal option and requires just one bundle of kale with sea salt and olive oil (coconut oil or avocado oil can also be used.

- 3 cups of raw kale pieces, cut from a fresh bundle, into bite-sized portions
- Sea salt or pink Himalayan salt
- Olive oil (coconut oil or avocado oil are also options)

Lightly and evenly coat all the kale pieces with olive oil and place them on a baking tray. Parchment paper is recommended to ensure the kale does not stick to the tray when baking in the oven.

Sprinkle evenly and lightly with sea salt over the chips, then bake for 8-10 minutes at 375 degrees. Keep an eye on the oven for the first one or two attempts of this recipe. Due to the type of kale (curly, red, etc.), the cooking time may be more or less by a minute or two, and may burn quickly or not cook fully (this can change within just one minute, as kale is thin and cooks fast!).

There are a few options and variations to consider for kale chips if you want to add a twist to the flavor:

Cumin or Curry Flavored Kale Chips

Add a sprinkle of curry powder and/or cumin mixed with sea salt. The baking time should be approximately the same time frame as the regular recipe.

Parmesan Kale Chips

Add a light coating of dried, shredded parmesan cheese along with the sea salt. Black pepper is also a good option combined with the parmesan and salt. These chips may take another one or two minutes to cook fully, approximately 10-12 minutes, at a temperature of 375 degrees.

Spicy Kale Chips

Combining a dash of chili powder, cayenne pepper or Cajun spice is ideal for spicy kale chips. These will cook for about 8-10 minutes, roughly the same time frame as the regular chips.

Baked Onion Rings

These are a nice alternative to the deep-fried variety, which is full of trans fats and unhealthy ingredients. This recipe is easily made with several ingredients to coat the onion rings and bake them for 15-16 minutes in the oven at 350 degrees.

- 2 medium or 1 large red onion, sliced into rings
- 1 cup of almond flour
- 2 eggs
- Sea salt
- Cajun spice
- Black pepper

Mix the black pepper, sea salt, and Cajun spice in a bowl, then combine with the almond flour. This will serve as the coating on the onion rings. Whisk the two eggs in a separate bowl, and coat each onion ring thoroughly first, before coating with the almond and spice combination, and place on a prepared baking tray. Bake for approximately 15-16 minutes, until the onion rings are crispy, but not burnt. Serve with salsa or coconut-based sour cream dip or enjoy as is. These are an excellent snack in place of potato chips or popcorn.

Spicy Guacamole

*A*vocados are a great option for the Paleo diet, as they are high in fiber, healthy fats, and energy. Guacamole is a great side or dish to include with a variety of meals, as a side to chili or skillet meal, or as a burger topping.

- 2 avocadoes, ripe
- Olive oil, about 2 teaspoons
- Freshly squeezed lime juice
- Chili powder or cayenne
- Grated onion, about 2 tablespoons

- ½ a tomato, diced
- Black pepper and sea salt
- Fresh cilantro

Mash the fresh avocados in a bowl and add in the sea salt, black pepper, olive oil, lime juice, and spices. Combine well, and fold in the tomatoes and onions, ensuring they are mixed well. Top with cilantro to serve.

FREQUENTLY ASKED QUESTIONS

ONCE YOU BEGIN ADAPTING to the Paleo diet, you may have additional questions or concerns that can be addressed here. The following frequently asked questions provide more information on how to approach individual situations and customizing your way of eating Paleo.

Question: Can the Paleo diet be adapted for vegan and plant-based diets?

Answer: The Paleo diet can be adapted to fit a plant-based meal plan. However, there are key vegan foods that would not be Paleo friendlies, such as soy, edamame beans, legumes, and fermented versions of soy, such as miso and tempeh. Dairy products would be replaced with nut-based milk, yogurt, and butter, made from almond, peanut, cashews and coconut milk. Plant-based proteins appropriate for the Paleo diet include nuts, seeds, dark greens, and sea vegetables. It may be a challenge to incorporate Paleo into a vegan diet, though with adequate research and dedication, it is possible.

Question: Is there a limitation on the amount of sugar you can have when following the Paleo diet?

Answer: Sugar is not strictly forbidden or avoided, as long as it is fructose or another natural, unrefined source, such as agave or maple syrup. As long as your diet and food choices are predominantly natural and without processing, including meat and dairy products in their natural, unflavored form, there will be little concern for excessive sugar, as you will only receive the required amounts in each serving. In other words, eating a fully natural, organic diet provides a balance of all nutrients on its own, without the need to strictly monitor sugar.

Question: Are there any drawbacks to following a Paleo diet?

Answer: Generally, there are no risks in following a Paleo diet, as all the foods are natural and full of nutrients, without any processed or artificial ingredients. There have been some concerns about the chances of increasing the risk of heart disease, due to the number of fats in the Paleo diet, though there are no studies to support this concern, and in fact, Paleo has shown a positive impact on heart health and reducing the risk of heart conditions, due to the number of nutrients and fiber, and the lack of processed foods. Choosing this way of eating will significantly reduce your risk of many diseases and conditions associated with unhealthy food choices.

Question: Is dairy allowed on the paleo diet?

Answer: On a strict paleo diet, dairy is not included; however, some people may add it in small amounts. Some Paleo diets allow for milk, cheese, yogurt, and butter if they are from grass-fed animals, though generally it's limited or avoided. It's important to determine how much dairy you want to include, if at all, and check the source to confirm how likely it is to be a good option. Grass-fed is ideal and should be the standard for meat products as well. If you can access raw, unpasteurized milk, some Paleo diets accept this as an option because it is unprocessed, and the goal of this diet is to include whole foods as much as possible. Depending on where you live, unpasteurized milk may or may not be available, depending on the food guidelines and legislation in your region. If you want to add dairy, and are unable to find unpasteurized as an option, there are grass-fed milk products available in natural food stores as a good option.

Question: Is Paleo similar to the keto diet?

Answer: There are some similarities between keto and Paleo, where the level of protein is moderate, and healthy fats are included in place of high carb, processed foods. There are some important differences as well:

- The keto or ketogenic diet focuses on adjusting the fat content to be high, around 75% of the diet, followed by moderate amounts of protein and low levels of carbohydrates. On the other hand, Paleo doesn't follow strict guidelines for how much of each macronutrient to include, but rather, focuses on the types of foods and nutrient quality instead.
- The paleo diet includes many of the same types of foods as Paleo, without being specific in fat and protein content. While the focus of both diets interns of ow foods are chosen is different, the outcome is generally the same for weight loss and overall results.
- Both diets focus on including healthy sources of protein, either meat or plant-based, preferably from organic and grass-fed sources. While the Paleo diet doesn't actively include dairy products, except for grass-fed and unpasteurized options, the keto diet allows for more full-

fat dairy products, provided they do not contain additives, flavors, and sugars.

Question: How long does it take to see the results of a Paleo diet?

Answer: Like any new way of eating, it can take a few weeks to one month to notice a change. Paleo is a lifestyle approach to eating, focusing on the quality of food choices you make, rather than focusing on portions and restrictions. To see the results of the diet, keep your meals planning and indulges consistent with natural, whole foods, and avoid all processed options. If you add in a few grains or a dish with non-Paleo food now and again, it's understandable, especially if they were regular choices in your meals before beginning this way of eating. Take your time, and don't feel discouraged if you don't see the results you expect right away. For most people, results take about one or two months, though it can happen sooner. Overall, you will reap the benefits of eating and feeling better.

Question: What is the purpose of the Paleo diet, and why was it developed?

Answer: The Paleo diet was developed to return to a primal way of eating, which does not include foods that are the result of farming or processing. It is strongly believed that our way of eating and health fares much better with the hunting and gathering method, which is most compatible with our development and genetics. Removing foods from our diet that involve farming and processing, is how we can realign our march to an original diet. This can alleviate many of the health conditions and problems we face today, which can be avoided by eating primal.

Question: Is the Paleo diet one of the best ways to eat?

Answer: It is considered one of the healthiest ways to eat because it closely follows the way our ancestors ate, which is based on natural meats, fruits, vegetables, nuts, and seeds. It doesn't restrict calories or require fasting, two factors that can affect some people's physical reactions to the diet. Following a balanced, nutritious way of eating is one of the best ways to eat, which Paleo aims to achieve.

Question: Can I follow the Paleo diet, even if I have allergies or serious reactions to certain types of foods contained in the Paleo diet?

Answer: Yes, anyone can follow the Paleo diet, and any foods that cause a reaction can simply be avoided. Often, the foods that create allergic reactions are processed foods, dairy, or wheat products, all of which are not included in the Paleo diet, except for some unpasteurized milk products. Shellfish and nut allergies can be avoided by omitting these foods completely. Fortunately, Paleo can be customized to give you a lot of options, which include a wide range of fruits and vegetables.

Question: Are there restaurants that cater specifically to the Paleo diet?

Answer: With the increase in popularity, there are some diners and restaurants that offer a good variety of Paleo-friendly foods, or they may be open to modifying menu choices to accommodate them. In urban areas, you may find more specific niche cafes and food services for certain dietary needs, many of which can fit within Paleo, such as gluten-free, ketogenic, and grass-fed meat options. Some cafes offer take-out services and custom orders that fit within a wide range of dietary options, including Paleo.

Question: Do people generally follow a Paleo diet for the long term?

Answer: It varies depending on your individual goals, though most people can easily adapt to Paleo for many years. It is sustainable,

PALEO DIET FOR BEGINNERS

includes food choices that are easy to find at grocery stores and markets. Once you notice and experience the advantages of the Paleo diet, you'll want to continue following it longer, as it can only make a positive impact on your life!

The Paleo diet is a way of eating that has captured the attention of many people worldwide, due to its many advantages and focus on nutrients. By enjoying a wide range of fresh fruits, vegetables, and lean meats, among many other food options, such as nuts and seeds, your body and health will reap the many benefits associated with good food choices and a sustainable, long-term lifestyle of eating and living well.

CONCLUSION

Tips, Suggestions for Success on the Paleo Diet

Now that you've begun your journey to living and eating the Paleo way of life, you will likely encounter situations where you're unsure of which foods items should be included. While the parameters are clear initially, many food options in stores are vague about their contents and hide as much about artificial ingredients and hidden sugars as they can. This raises a lot of concerns, especially when avoiding as many unnatural and unhealthy options as possible. To ensure your success on this diet, consider the following tips and suggestions:

- Choose fresh produce only, and shop for frozen in a natural state, where the fresh option of fruits and/or vegetables is not readily available. Frozen vegetables and fruits are a great alternative when the option you want is not in season or not available in the produce section. Avoid canned fruits, as they contain syrup and sugars, while canned vegetables and related sauces contain high sodium, and other artificial ingredients, including sugar.

- Meat and dairy quality are more important than quantity. Make the most of your neighborhood, and locate local butchers, farmer's markets and shops that provide good options. Some supermarkets offer local goods reflecting the community and may offer organic meats and/or cheese options in their deli. Choose fresh or frozen meats, and avoid processed meat slices, as they contain carcinogens and nitrates, both of which contribute to a higher risk or cancer and heart disease.

- Nuts and seeds tend to be expensive, especially if they are fresh and from a good source. If possible, buy in bulk, so that you can choose the portion and custom the types of nuts and seeds you prefer. Cashew and pistachios tend to be expensive, whereas walnuts, peanuts, almonds, and pecans are less costly.

- Create as many foods and meals from home as possible. There are plenty of grocery stores and restaurants that offer Paleo-friendly foods, which is helpful in a pinch and convenient. However, some store-bought items may not be as fitting within the Paleo diet as they claim. For this reason, read labels and ingredients on all the items before you purchase them, and beware of any claims that are not accurate. Save your wallet and your diet by knowing what to buy.

KETO DIET

FOR BEGINNERS

A Guide for Losing Weight. Live the
Keto Lifestyle

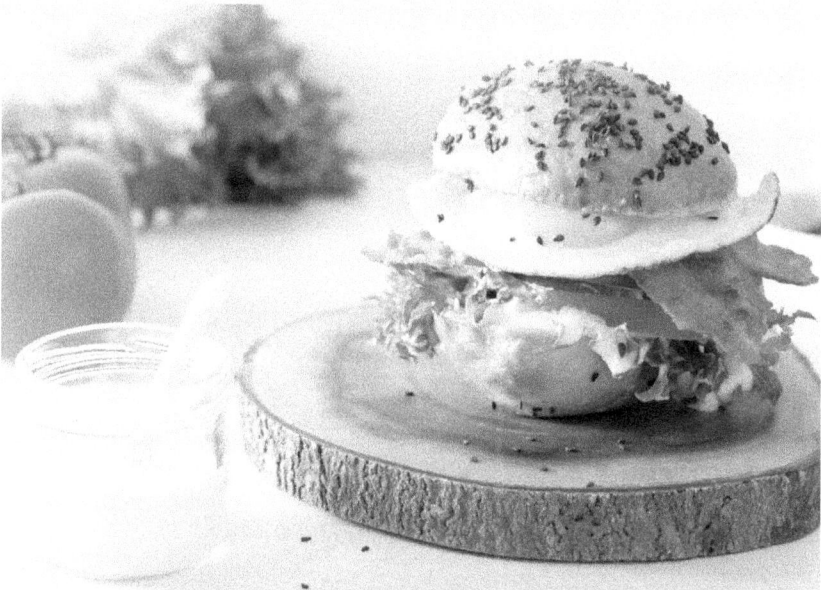

Cindy Chen

INTRODUCTION

Before anybody commits to a ketogenic diet, it is important to learn about what it actually is you can determine whether or not this diet suits your needs and is healthy for your individual body. Many people with health problems jump into a keto diet without fully understanding what it is only to create more health problems for themselves.

What Is a Ketogenic Diet?

A Ketogenic Diet, or a Keto diet is a specific diet that involves eating certain foods and eliminating others. This is done in this specific case in an effort to induce a state of ketosis all of the time in one's body. We will look at what Ketosis is below.

Ketosis

Ketosis is a state that the body enters when there is a lack of recently-ingested sugars (carbohydrates) or stored sugars, and it must instead use stored fat to get its energy. When the body enters this state, it breaks down its fat stores and the breakdown of these fat stores creates an acid as a by-product. This acid that is created is called a *Ketone*. When in a state of ketosis, the brain is able to use ketones for energy instead of carbohydrates or sugars like it normally would.

This state of ketosis in the brain has many benefits for the brain cells. The way that this works is that the Ketones in the brain signal to the brain cells that there are low levels of energy sources, which is why the brain begins using ketones for energy. It is not completely understood much further than this as of yet, but ketosis in the brain has produced many positive effects for the brain like the protection of brain cells. This leads to a reduction in the likelihood of diseases like Alzheimer's or Parkinson's.

The ketones produced from the breakdown of fat stores are released in urine and this is how you can tell when your body is in a state of ketosis. It is beneficial to know when you are in this state if you are attempting to get your body to break down fat stores, knowing that this is the state you are in you then know that your methods are functioning. If you are interested, you can test this using test strips which will tell you the acidity of your urine. The more acidic in your urine, the higher presence of ketones.

The Ketogenic Diet

The Keto diet involves eating very high-fat and low-carb (or no carb) foods. In terms of carbs, in a Keto diet, they are restricted to 10% or less of your total daily caloric intake. This works out to somewhere around 50 grams of carbohydrates. Protein will contribute about 20 or 30 percent of your daily caloric intake.

When it comes to fats, there are different types. Many people refer to them as "good" and "bad" fats. But we will instead call them healthy fats and unhealthy fats. Most of the time, when you think of fats, you likely think of fried foods and packaged baked goods.

There are many other foods, however, that contain the healthy types of fats.

The way that this diet works is that it eliminates the carbohydrates that you would normally eat to give you energy throughout the day so that your body has to turn to other sources of energy. This puts your body in a state of ketosis (hence the name).

Plant-based Option of the Ketogenic Diet

With plant-based alternatives on the rise in our modern society, it is important to know that people that prefer plant-based foods can still take on the ketogenic diet. However, the term 'plant-based' diet isn't exactly what you may think it means. A plant-based diet is focused on only plant-forward sources of food. This is not only restricted to vegetables and fruits, but any other plant sources of food as well. This diet does not mean the same thing as being vegetarian or vegan, and it does not say anything about what you can eat in terms of meat and dairy. However, there are many similarities to a vegetarian diet or a Mediterranean diet. A Mediterranean diet comes from the foods that would commonly be eaten by people who reside around the Mediterranean; thus, it includes foods that would be grown and found in these regions. Many of these foods are plant-based, but it also includes fish, poultry and dairy in small quantities. This is one example of a diet that is mostly plant-based. A vegetarian diet is another example of a diet that can be mostly plant-based, but without including meats. However, a vegetarian diet is not always plant-based if the individual eats a high amount of processed foods.

The plant-based diet can be flexible and tailored to the specific individual, which is one of its benefits. This diet is focused on keeping foods as natural as possible and avoiding heavily processed foods.

THE KETOGENIC DIET

LET's begin learning about some of the benefits of following a ketogenic diet, the best foods to eat in this diet, plant-based alternatives and the pros and cons of the keto diet. Again, this is important as learning about the details of the keto diet will help you determine if this is suitable for your specific health needs. Keep in mind that if you are unsure of whether or not the keto diet is good or sustainable for you, seek advice from a health and dietary professional.

Benefits of the Keto Diet

The Keto diet comes with a number of benefits, some of which we have seen in the introduction to this book. Here, we will examine the benefits in a little more detail.

1. Autophagy and Brain Health

*A*s I briefly mentioned in the introduction, the Keto diet has been shown to be very beneficial for the brain cells. This is because of something called Autophagy. Autophagy is a process that the body uses to clean itself out. This process involves small "hunter" particles that go around the cells of your body looking for cell components that are old and damaged. The hunter particles then take these cell components apart, getting rid of the damaged parts and saving the useful parts to make new cells later. These hunter cells can also use leftover useful parts to create energy for the body. The benefits of this process are far-reaching. This leads to a clean and efficient environment within the cells of your body and keeps everything functioning well. It also reduces the risk of diseases like cancer. When you are eating according to the Keto diet, the state of Ketosis that it leads to actually acts as a signal for Autophagy in the brain. This cleans the brain cells and keeps them healthy. This process reduces your risk of cancers in the brain or diseases of the brain like Alzheimer's. Eating according to a Keto diet is not only beneficial for the body, as we will see, but it is also beneficial for the mind. Aside from preventing disease, it helps to keep your brain sharp and functioning well.

1. Skin Health

*A*s you likely know, skin health can be closely related to diet and sugar intake. The Keto diet reduces carbohydrates and sugars; it can lead to decreased levels of acne and improved overall skin health. This is because ingesting high levels of sugar leads to dramatic rises and dips in blood sugar levels which affects the health of a person's skin.

1. Cancer

*W*e previously discussed how the Keto diet could lead to a decreased risk of brain cancer, but it can also reduce your risk of other cancers. Similar to how we discussed that Autophagy cleans out the cells of the body, it does this in other parts of the body and not just in the brain. When it does this, it can clean out cells that could become cancerous, or cells that are already cancerous and thus, it can prevent many different types of cancer. It has also been shown to be an effective treatment for cancer along with chemotherapy and radiation. Further, the stabilizing effects that this diet has on blood sugar levels can also reduce the risk of some cancers that have been associated with blood sugar regulation complications.

1. Heart Health

*I*f the Keto diet consists of healthy fats and not only fats from animal sources (we will look at this more later), it can lead to better heart health. This is because it can actually reduce cholesterol levels.

1. Seizures

*I*n people who suffer from epilepsy, the presence of ketones during ketosis as a result of the Keto diet can reduce seizures. This has been shown to be effective in children suffering from this disease.

1. PCOS

*P*COS or Polycystic Ovarian Syndrome is something that many women suffer from. This disease leads women's ovaries to develop cysts which can lead to very painful periods, weight gain and infertility. It has been shown that a diet high in carbohydrates can negatively affect this disease and exacerbate symptoms. By following the Keto diet, showed improvement in the general health of women with PCOS, reduced their symptoms (including leading to weight loss) and helped to mitigate the progression of the disease.

*B*est Foods to Eat on a Keto Diet

*Y*ou may be wondering what types of foods you are able to eat on a keto diet. As a reminder, in general, the Ketogenic diet involves eating very high-fat and low-carb (or no carb) foods. In terms of carbs, in a Keto diet, they are restricted to 10% or less of your total daily caloric intake. This works out to somewhere around 50 grams of carbohydrates. Protein will contribute about 20 or 30 percent of your daily caloric intake. We will look at some examples of the foods that are included in a Ketogenic diet in this section.

*F*ish is a great way to get healthy fats when following a Keto diet. Certain fish are very low in carbohydrates but high in good fats, making them perfect for this diet. They also contain minerals and vitamins that will be good for your health. Salmon is a great fish to eat on this diet as it is essentially carbohydrate-free. Many fish also include essential fatty acids that we can only get through our diet. Other fish that are good to eat on a Keto diet are;

- Sardines
- Mackerel
- Herring
- Trout
- Albacore Tuna

*S*hellfish are also a good choice, though some of them contain small amounts of carbohydrates, so it is important to keep this in mind when including them in a Keto diet. The following shellfish are arranged in order of increasing carbohydrate content. They range from 3 grams to 7 grams of carbohydrates per 100-gram serving.

- Squid
- Oysters
- Octopus
- Clams
- Mussels

*V*egetables are included in a Keto diet, as they contain low numbers of calories and carbohydrates but have many beneficial vitamins and minerals. The body does not digest fiber, so it is good to eat vegetables that contain fiber as they help you to feel full without actually filling your body with digestible carbohydrates. When looking at which vegetables to eat, take the total amount of carbohydrates and subtract from it the amount of fiber to find out how many carbs your body will actually absorb from it. Some examples of fibrous vegetables include the following;

- Celery
- Spinach
- Brussels Sprouts
- Asparagus
- Bok Choy
- Cabbage
- Green Beans
- Artichokes

Some vegetables, however, include high amounts of carbohydrates. These vegetables include starchy vegetables such as root vegetables. You must be careful when including these vegetables in a Keto diet since they are not too high in fiber but contain a high starch content.

- Potatoes
- Beets
- Yams
- Squash

Cheese may surprise you as a good choice in a diet plan, but it is great for the Ketogenic diet as it contains high fat content but very low carb content, and this is true for all types of cheese. Cheese has also been shown to protect against heart disease in some studies as well as help with fat loss and body composition improvements.

- Cheddar cheese
- Ricotta cheese
- Swiss cheese
- Parmigiano Reggiano
- Feta cheese

*A*vocados are a great option for healthy fat for anyone, especially those on a Ketogenic diet. Avocados are high in fiber so their carbohydrate content is reduced to only about two grams of carbohydrates per 100-gram serving. They are high in healthy fats at the same time, so they are the ideal Keto food. They also contain vitamins and minerals that are healthy for improved overall health. Avocados have been shown to reduce "bad" cholesterol and improve "good" cholesterol.

*M*eat and Poultry make up a large part of a Ketogenic diet. Meats and poultry that are fresh and not processed do not include any carbohydrates, but contain high levels of protein. Eating lean meats when on a low-carbohydrate diet helps to maintain your strength and muscle mass that could otherwise decrease as a result of decreased carbohydrate intake. Grass-fed meats, in particular, are rich in antioxidants and beneficial fats, which is great for a Ketogenic diet.

· · ·

*E*ggs are another amazing Ketogenic food. They have virtually no carbohydrates and contain protein. Eggs help you to feel full for longer and keep blood sugar levels consistent, which is great for overall health. The whole egg is good for you, as the yolk is where the nutrients are. The cholesterol found within egg yolks also has been shown to reduce the risk of heart disease, despite what most people think. When on a Keto diet, do not be afraid of the yolk of the egg.

*T*here are numerous oils that you can find on the shelves of any grocery store. Knowing which to choose can be difficult. In this section, we will look at the best oils for a Ketogenic diet. The following oils are known to be good sources of healthy fats;

- Coconut Oil- This oil is extremely versatile and can be used in cooking, for skincare, in coffee and so on. Coconut oil specifically has been shown to increase ketosis in the brain. Coconut oil can also lead to prolonged states of ketosis which extends the benefits over a longer term.
- Olive Oil- olive oil is great for reducing inflammation, and it is carbohydrate-free
- Avocado Oil

*J*ust as olive oil is good for the Keto diet, so are **olives.** They have the same benefits of olive oil, but in solid form instead. Since you would not enjoy drinking olive oil, eating olives is a great way to get these benefits in a quick, snack form.

*G*reek Yogurt is a food that is high in protein but small amounts of carbohydrates.

*C*ottage Cheese is another similar food that contains high protein and low carbohydrates. They both help you to feel full, from eating small amounts and keep you full for longer because of the protein they contain, which keeps giving you energy for a prolonged period. These can be put together with other foods or eaten alone.

*N*uts and **Seeds** are foods that are high in fat and fiber, and low in carbohydrates. The carbohydrate count varies among nuts and seeds, but those with the lowest levels of carbohydrates are below. All of the following include between 0 and 3 grams of carbohydrates;

- Brazil Nuts
- Pecans
- Walnuts
- Flaxseeds
- Chia Seeds
- Macadamia nuts
- Sesame seeds
- Almonds

*B*erries are different from other fruits in that they are low in carbohydrates. Most fruits are high in carbohydrates because of the sugars they contain, but berries are an exception. They are high in fiber and very low in carbohydrates. In particular, **raspberries** and **blackberries** have the same amount of digestible carbohydrates as fiber, making them very healthy. Berries also contain many healthy antioxidants and anti-inflammatory compounds. Other berries include **blueberries** and **strawberries.**

*B*utter is a food that is high in fat but low in carbohydrates (virtually zero). This is also true for **cream.** Cream and butter have been shown to promote fat loss and reduce the risk of stroke and heart attack.

*C*offee and **tea** are fine to consume on a Keto dict, but they must be unsweetened. These drinks on their own contain no calories or carbohydrates, but they are healthy because of their antioxidants and their influence on the body's metabolism. Teas like green tea and black tea are especially good for the body's metabolism. It is fine to add cream to coffee or tea on the Ketogenic diet, but only cream and not low-fat milk as it contains sugar.

*C*ocoa is a superfood, which is why it is included in this list. Cocoa and dark chocolate are rich in nutrients like antioxidants and has been shown to reduce the risk of diseases like high blood pressure, heart disease and stroke. When choosing dark chocolate, it is important to pick one that is unsweetened and no less than 70% cocoa so that there are not too many carbohydrates contained within.

*I*n a Ketogenic diet, it is important to choose the carbohydrates you will include wisely, as there is not much room to include them. Choose food sources that are not very carbohydrate-dense and that include other beneficial nutrients. Some people on a keto diet also choose to supplement Ketones, which can help to get your body into a state of ketosis quicker and can help you to feel the benefits of the mental sharpness that

*P*lant-based Alternative for the Ketogenic Diet

*F*ruits are included in a plant-based diet, as they are naturally-occurring in nature.

*E*xamples of fruits that you can eat include the following;

- Citrus fruits such as oranges, grapefruits, lemons, and limes
- Melons of a variety of sorts
- Apples
- Bananas
- Berries including strawberries, blueberries, blackberries, raspberries and so on
- Grapes

*V*egetables are a great source of energy and nutrients and they include a wide range of naturally-occurring vivid colors that should all be included in your diet.

- Carrots
- Broccoli and cauliflower
- Asparagus
- Kale
- All sorts of peppers including hot peppers, bell peppers
- Tomatoes
- Root vegetables (that are a good source of healthy, complete carbohydrates) such as potatoes, sweet potatoes, all types of squash, and beets.

*F*ruits and vegetables aren't the only types of foods that you can eat on a plant-based diet. There are a variety of other plant-based foods that are included.

*L*egumes are a great source of protein as well as fiber, and there are many different types to choose from. These include the following;

- All sorts of beans including black beans, green beans, and kidney beans
- Peas
- Lentils of all colors
- Chickpeas
- Peas

*S*eeds are another great source of nutrients, vitamins, and minerals, and they are very versatile. These include the following;

- Sesame seeds
- Pumpkin seeds
- Sunflower seeds
- Hemp, flax and chia seeds are all especially good for your health

*N*uts are a great way to get protein if you are choosing not to eat meat or if you are vegan. They also are packed with nutrients. Some examples are below.

- Almonds
- Brazil Nuts
- Cashews
- Macadamia nuts
- Pistachios
- Pecans

*T*here are some **healthy fats** that are essential components of any person's diet, as the beneficial compounds that they contain cannot be made by our bodies; thus, we rely solely on or diet to get them. These compounds are Omega-3 Fatty Acids, monounsaturated and polyunsaturated fats. Below are some healthy sources of these compounds;

- Avocados
- Healthy, plant-based oils including olive oil and canola oil
- Hemp, chia and flax seeds
- Walnuts

When it comes to carbohydrates, these should be consumed in the form of **whole grains**, as they are high in fiber, which will help to prevent overeating. Whole grains also include essential minerals- those that we can only get from our diet just like those essential compounds found in healthy fats. These essential minerals are selenium, magnesium and copper. Sources of these whole grains include the following;

- Quinoa
- Rye, Barley, buckwheat
- Whole grain oats
- Brown rice
- Whole grain bread can be hard to find these days in the grocery store, as many brown breads disguise themselves as whole grain when, in fact, they are not. However, there are whole grain breads if you take the time to look at the ingredients list.

Plant-Based milk is another way to eat plant-based while having things that require milk or a milk-like substance. These are great if you are dairy-free or vegan, or if you simply prefer to get your milk from a plant source instead of an animal source. Be sure to check the ingredients to see if there are any added chemicals or sugars and try to choose the most natural. Some examples of these include the following;

- Rice milk
- Hemp milk
- Coconut milk
- Almond milk
- Oat milk
- Soy milk

Raw Diet Vs. Cooked Food Diet

Before closing this chapter, we are going to discuss something that is heavily debated within the diet and nutrition world. Raw versus cooked food. There are some people who are strongly committed to the idea that raw food is better for your diet than cooked food. Raw food includes food that is unprocessed, unheated, uncooked, and fermented.

Benefits of a Raw Diet

People of these beliefs believe the following points;

1. Vitamins

When you cook your food, some of the nutrients that

the food contained when it was raw may not be present anymore when cooked. Specifically, this can happen with a number of vitamins. This is due to the fact that some vitamins are water-soluble, meaning that they dissolve in water, so if you are boiling a vegetable for example, the vitamins from the food may dissolve in the water and exit the food itself. Water-soluble vitamins include vitamin C, and B vitamins. The majority of the vitamins that are lost during cooking will be those that are water soluble, but some others like Vitamin A and some minerals may also be lost or deactivated through cooking, but to a much lesser degree. Since boiling vegetables can cause them to lose vitamins, a possible solution could be to cook them in a different manner such as through roasting, steaming or frying them. This will lead to less vitamin loss as these methods use much less water. Another possible solution could be boiling a vegetable for less time, as this will result in less nutrient loss.

1. Enzymes

The other thing that is believed by raw foodists (those who consume a raw diet) is that during the process of cooking food, many enzymes that are contained within are denatured because of the heat. These enzymes can aid your gut in digestion, but if they are denatured, it will require more enzyme recruitment within your gut to break down the food. Raw foodists believe that this ends up putting long-term stress on your digestive system. While it is true that enzymes become denatured at high heat levels, there is little scientific evidence that this causes any undue stress on the body.

1. Toxicity

*S*ome extreme raw foodists believe that a cooked food diet is actually unhealthy and that it is actually toxic for the human body.

*D*rawbacks of a Raw Diet

On the other hand, though, there are some drawbacks that are worth noting when considering a raw food diet.

1. Vitamins

*W*hile it is true that some vitamins are destroyed during the cooking process of food, there are others, however, that are more readily available for your body to use when your food is cooked.

1. Challenging

*I*t is quite difficult to follow a complete or even 70% raw food diet. It is rare that a person will be able to stick to a raw diet on a long-term basis.

1. Bacteria and Illness

*W*hen it comes to raw foods, some can be dangerous to consume. There are some bacteria that are present in foods that are killed during the cooking process, which is why meats like poultry or pork must be cooked to a very specific minimum internal temperature for them to be safe to consume. This is a risk that is taken if a person wants to eat a raw food diet that still contains meats or fish, but if they are eating a raw vegan diet, it is less of a concern.

1. Chewing

*Y*ou may not know this, but digestion actually begins in the mouth. The first step of digestion is when you chew your food. Cooking your food makes this first step easier, and eating raw food can make it more difficult to chew, resulting in tougher digestion and more stress on the gut later on in the digestion process. If the food is in bigger pieces or not properly chewed when it reaches the gut, it can result in painful gas and bloating. Also, if you are able to chew your raw food thoroughly, it usually takes much more energy and effort to do so. This is especially true for meats, as they are tough and difficult to chew if they are uncooked.

1. Anti-Nutrients

*T*here is something called an anti-nutrient that is found within some legumes, beans and grains. Anti-nutrients are something that, when ingested, prevent the body from absorbing nutrients from the foods that contain them. When you cook these foods though, the number and effectiveness of anti-nutrients become greatly reduced, allowing your body to absorb more nutrients from the food.

1. Antioxidants

KETO DIET FOR BEGINNERS

*I*n some vegetables, their antioxidants are made more readily available to your body by cooking the vegetables, so by eating them raw, your body will be unable to extract and absorb these antioxidants. These antioxidants have been shown to reduce the risk of certain cancers and heart disease.

1. Pleasant Aroma and Appearance

*C*ooked food, in general, has a much more pleasant aroma and appearance than uncooked food. The first part of eating happens with your eyes and your nose. When you see and smell cooked food, your mouth begins to water and your digestive system begins to prepare for the food to be ingested, leading to more effective digestion.

*T*he nutrients and vitamins that a person's body can get from food are completely dependent on the body's ability to digest the food, as this is how the body gets nutrients from the food. Without proper digestion, the body is unable to extract the nutrients it needs. Thus, it is important to make an informed decision about whether to eat your food cooked or uncooked depending on the ease with which it can be chewed and digested in addition to the scientific research about the availability of its nutrients and vitamins.

*F*urther, you must examine some foods' personal benefits and drawbacks when it comes to cooking or eating them raw. For example, tomatoes lose some of their vitamin C content when you cook them, but their antioxidant content increases. Thus, you must make a personal decision about which you would prefer or which you need most at this stage of your life.

*I*n some cases, there are foods that are better for your health, either raw or cooked. These foods and their preferred method of consumption are listed below;

- Broccoli is much healthier for the human body when consumed raw. This is because there is a compound contained within it that has proven to be cancer-fighting, but that is found in much smaller quantities in cooked broccoli.

- Onions are beneficial for the health of your blood when consumed raw. Raw onions lead to less blood clotting, but cooking them leads this benefit to be greatly reduced.

- Cabbage, when cooked for a long period of time, loses its beneficial enzyme for cancer prevention. Eating cabbage raw or only lightly cooked maintains much of this benefit.

- Garlic has anti-cancer benefits when it is eaten raw, but when cooked, this benefit is denatured.

- Mushrooms have been found to contain a compound that could be a carcinogen for humans. By cooking them, you are breaking down this compound and eliminating its possible harmful effects. Cooking them also releases an antioxidant that is inactive when they are raw.

- Asparagus contains many vitamins, but they are inaccessible when it is raw because the stem is so fibrous that it is difficult for the body to digest it enough to absorb these nutrients. Coking it breaks the stem down enough for the vitamins to be released and absorbed during digestion.

- Spinach contains many elements like zinc, calcium, and magnesium, but they are made much more available when it is cooked.

*A*s you can see in the list above, there are some cases where you may prefer certain methods of preparation for certain foods. Keeping this in mind, a diet that is comprised of a mix of raw and cooked foods may be the most beneficial for most humans.

*N*utrients Needed for a Healthy Ketogenic Diet

. . .

*W*e have discussed briefly some of the nutrients that are found in certain vegetables and foods through our discussion of which foods are included in the Keto diet (with plant-based alternatives suggested as well). In this section, we are going to look at the most beneficial nutrients for your body and where/ how you can find them when following a specific diet.

*O*mega 3 Fatty Acids

*O*mega-3 Fatty Acids are fats that are needed in your diet as the body cannot make them on its own. These fatty acids are a certain type in a list of other fatty acids, but this type (Omega-3) are the most essential and the most beneficial for our brains and bodies in general. They have numerous effects on the brain, including reducing inflammation (which reduces the risk of Alzheimer's) and maintaining and improving mood and cognitive function, including specifically memory. Omega-3's have these greatly beneficial effects because of the way that they act in the brain, which is what makes them so essential to our diets. Omega-3 Fatty Acids increase the production of new nerve cells in the brain by acting specifically on the nerve stem cells within the brain, causing new and healthy nerve cells to be generated.

*O*mega-3 fatty acids can be found in fish like salmon, sardines, black cod, and herring. It can also be taken as a pill-form supplement for those who do not eat fish or cannot eat enough of it. It can also be taken in the form of a fish oil supplement like krill oil.

. . .

*O*mega-3's are by far the most important nutrient that you need to ensure you are ingesting because of the numerous benefits that come from it, both in the brain and in the rest of the body. While supplements are often the last step when it comes to trying to include something in your diet, for Omega-3's the benefits are too great to potentially miss by trying to receive all of it from your diet.

*S*ulphoraphane

*B*russels Sprouts, Cabbage, Kale, Broccoli Sprouts have in common? All of these green vegetables have one thing in common- they all contain Sulforaphane. Sulforaphane is a plant chemical that is found naturally in these vegetables. This is an antioxidant that acts in a similar way to turmeric and thus has similar benefits. Sulforaphane like turmeric, induces autophagy in the brain which helps to reduce the risk of Alzheimer's, Parkinson's and dementia which are all neurodegenerative diseases. *Neurodegenerative* means that the cells in the brain called nerves are damaged and broken down, which leads to cognitive decline like Alzheimer's or physical decline as in Parkinson's. These vegetables can help to treat these diseases by slowing their progression, as they are all diseases that come about over time. There is no cure yet, but the treatment at this stage involves delaying the progression of these diseases.

. . .

*S*ulforaphane can be found in the aforementioned vegetables, but the strongest source is in broccoli sprouts. It can also be taken concentrated in a supplement form.

*C*alcium

*C*alcium is beneficial for the healthy circulation of blood, and for maintaining strong bones and teeth. Calcium can come from dairy products like milk, yogurt, and cheese. It can also be found in leafy greens like kale and broccoli and sardines.

*M*agnesium

*M*agnesium is beneficial for your diet, as it also helps you to maintain strong bones and teeth. Magnesium and Calcium are most effective when ingested together, as Magnesium helps in the absorption of calcium. It also helps to reduce migraines and is great for calmness and relieving anxiety. Magnesium can be found in leafy green vegetables like kale and spinach, as well as fruits like bananas and raspberries, legumes like beans and chickpeas, vegetables like peas, cabbage, green beans, asparagus and brussels sprouts, and fish like tuna and salmon.

*B*ioactive Compounds

. . .

*B*ioactive compounds are compounds found within foods that act in the body in beneficial ways. The bioactive compounds found within berries, such as Acai Berries, Strawberries, and Blueberries are very beneficial for your health. The bioactive compounds in these specific types of berries work in the brain to induce autophagy and reduce inflammation. This leads to the protection of brain cells in this case from *oxidative stress*. Oxidative stress is something that can happen within the brain when there is an imbalance of oxygen, which can cause reduced cognitive functioning. These berries and their induction of autophagy helps to reduce this by keeping the balance of oxygen at a healthy level.

WEIGHT LOSS USING THE KETO DIET

A KETOGENIC DIET is greatly beneficial in losing weight for those who can stick with it. Since more and more people who are plant-based now have decided to pursue the Keto diet as well, it is important that we take plant-based alternatives into consideration as we further explore the role that Keto plays in weight loss. There are benefits to both a plant-based diet and a ketogenic diet; their benefits combine to make a diet that is very beneficial for your health and your waistline.

We are going to delve into the specific ways that a Ketogenic diet can lead to rapid weight loss. First, though, we will discuss weight loss as a general concept. The most basic concept of weight loss is that you must put your body in a calorie deficit in order to lose weight. What this means is that you must eat fewer calories than you burn, which will result in a loss of weight. The equation for this concept is below;

The number of calories that you ingest – **(minus)** The number of calories you use to survive (for example, walking, eating, breathing) – **(minus)** The extra calories burned from exercise = **(equals)** = + **(positive)** or – **(negative)**

The number that results from this equation will be either positive or negative. If the number is positive, this means that you ingested more calories than you burned. If the number is negative, this means that you burned more calories than you ingested. If the number is zero, this means that calories ingested and calories burned are equal to one another. If the number is zero, this indicates "breaking even" in terms of your energy. If the number is positive, you can envision it like having more energy than you were able to use. When this occurs, the extra energy is stored as fat in the body. If the number is negative, you used more energy than you had and this translates to weight loss, as once the energy is all used up, the fat stores will begin to be used for additional energy.

How Does a Ketogenic Diet Help You Lose Weight?

The ketogenic diet helps you lose weight by combining four dietary fundamentals; hunger and satiety, water weight, fewer carbohydrates, autophagy and metabolism. This chapter will help you understand how these four fundamentals work together in a ketogenic diet to help you lose weight.

Hunger and Satiety

Any time you eat mostly plant-sourced foods or foods that are closer to their natural state, they will contain high amounts of fiber and large water content, especially in the case of vegetables. This means that people who eat a plant-based Keto diet will feel full earlier than those who do not and will remain full for longer. This is because of the high fiber and the high content of water, which fills a person's stomach much quicker than other foods would.

Vegetables have a very low-calorie content for their size, which means that they will fill your stomach without giving you a large calorie count. Because of this, when you become full from eating a salad, for example, you will not be able to eat any more food but you will not have ingested a large number of calories. This can lead to a calorie deficit and subsequent weight loss if this type of eating is continued.

Further, there have been studies that have shown following a keto-genic diet (high fat, low carb, moderate protein) leads to lower levels of ghrelin in the body. Ghrelin is a hormone that leads to feelings of hunger. By feeling less hungry overall and feeling fuller more quickly when you do eat, this will lead to a decrease in calo-ries consumed over the course of the day and a reduction in weight due to a calorie deficit.

Water Weight

Carbohydrates hold onto a lot of water. By greatly reducing your intake of carbohydrates, you are also reducing your intake of water. By also reducing the amount of stored carbohydrates, you are reducing your amount of stored water as well. When you begin eating according to the Keto diet, your body's stored carbohydrates are used for energy quite early on. At this point, you will see a reduction in weight because of the water that went along with these stores being used up.

Significantly Fewer Carbohydrates

By reducing the amount of carbohydrates you intake drastically, you will be reducing the amount of sugar that you intake drasti-cally as well. As we discussed previously, the more sugar you intake, the more blood sugar spikes you put your body through, which leads to an increase in stored fat. Because the blood sugar level spikes so drastically, your body releases a large amount of insulin to accommodate and it leads to fat storage as a result in order to combat the spike in blood sugar. This happens especially around the abdominal area. By switching to a diet that is low in carbohydrates and high in healthy fats, you are able to keep your insulin levels consistent, which will prevent your body from storing as much fat and will even encourage your body to use fat stores for energy instead of sugars. This diet leads to a quicker metabolism which means that the energy will be used up much quicker and more efficiently, reducing the chances of storing this energy for later. All of these things that happen as a result of reducing carbohydrate intake lead to weight loss.

Autophagy and Metabolism

As we discussed earlier, Autophagy is a large part of why the Ketogenic diet is so successful in terms of weight loss.

Metabolism is a large term that describes the breakdown of one thing in order to create energy. In more specific terms, it is all of the processes in the body that work together to maintain life. This happens when you eat food, and it is digested to absorb nutrients and create energy for your body to function. This also happens on a smaller level in each cell of the body by way of Autophagy, as it aids in the breakdown of old or damaged cell components, and this breakdown creates energy for the cell.

When the cells of your body are experiencing a lack of nutrition in the form of sugar, autophagy is triggered in order to create more energy for the cell to use by breaking down cell parts. Along with this, there is also a release of hormones by the body in an effort to use the energy that it is creating in the most efficient way possible. These hormones make the fat stores of the body more easily broken down and more accessible as a source of energy. Because of this, the body's rate of metabolism increases during these times of cellular starvation, and the body loses fat, resulting in weight loss. Therefore, the more often that your body is in a state of Ketosis, the more often this process of Autophagy will be occurring.

Using Ketogenic Diet to Help You Lose Weight Healthily

While eating, according to a diet, seems to promise many benefits, you must ensure that you are following the diet in a healthy way. With this diet in particular, it is important to ensure that you are drinking enough water. While it can be tempting to watch the pounds drop as your body loses water weight along with your decrease in carbohydrate intake, this can also leave you feeling dehydrated. Be sure to drink enough water so that you can combat the water lost through your carbohydrate stores and the lack of ingested water through the intake of carbohydrates.

Another point to note is that while you want to ensure you are at a calorie deficit in order to lose weight, this diet is not designed to keep you feeling hungry and as if you are starving yourself. Instead, you should feel satisfied and full enough simply due to the choices of foods that you are making. As I mentioned, vegetables are very low in calories for the amount of volume they occupy in your stomach, so this is a clear and effective way to avoid being left feeling hungry while still losing weight and getting all of your nutrients.

THE ROLE THAT KETO PLAYS IN DISEASE PREVENTION

❧

THROUGHOUT THIS BOOK, I have mentioned many times the many benefits of following a Ketogenic. Scientists and researches have found evidence that using a ketogenic diet can prevent diseases like cancer or heart disease. In this section, we will look into these benefits in more depth and how they work.

Autophagy Prevents Disease

One of the ways that this diet leads to the reduction of disease risk or can even act as a treatment for disease is because of Autophagy. Autophagy is a process that the body uses to clean itself out. This process involves small "hunter" particles that go around the cells of your body looking for cell components that are old and damaged. The hunter particles then take these cell components apart, getting rid of the damaged parts and saving the useful parts to make new cells later. These hunter cells can also use leftover useful parts to create energy for the body. There are certain environments that the cells must recognize in order for Autophagy to begin, and the Ketogenic diet is one of the ways that this environment can be achieved. As I mentioned, the Ketogenic diet puts the body in a state of Ketosis, as it leads the liver to produce Ketones. The cells of the body recognize this environment of Ketosis and in response, Autophagy is triggered. Therefore, eating according to a Ketogenic diet leads to the triggering of Autophagy which has countless benefits for the body and for disease prevention and treatment.

Autophagy Prevents General Illness

Autophagy plays a part in the immune system by killing infected cells before they can spread and infect other cells. By the process of Autophagy, the cell is able to be rid of the pathogens that have infected it without the need for a full immune system response (which would be very taxing for the body), depending on the level of infection in the body. The process of Autophagy is already occurring in our cells much of the time, and it has expanded its regular functioning in order to serve an extra purpose within the cell, which turns out to be greatly beneficial for our general health.

Autophagy Improve Lifespan

Autophagy is essential for the longevity of the organism- in this case, the human. Autophagy has been shown to have effects on aging and this is why it plays such an important role in lifespan. The reason for this is twofold. The first reason is that the cells that it acts in are often damaged or injured and by way of autophagy, the disease or virus that is attempting to infect the organism is unable to spread, allowing the organism to continue living a relatively healthy life. This type of disease control increases the longevity of the organism.

The second reason is that autophagy is essential to maintaining the health of specific tissues and organs, which keeps them running smoothly and functioning at their best, which is also another factor that influences lifespan. If the organs and tissues are healthy, the organism as a whole will be healthy and will keep living. In these two ways, autophagy plays a large role in the longevity and lifespan of the organisms and their cells.

Helps With Inflammation and Inflammatory Diseases

Inflammation is a reaction that occurs in the body in response to things such as pathogens or irritations. Inflammation is a response intended to protect us from whatever signaled the inflammation to occur. It does this by increasing the number of inflammatory cells in the area where the irritant or pathogen is located. The inflammatory cells are there to remove the irritant, promote new cell growth to replace cells that were damaged by the irritant and then to promote overall repair of the area. On the outside of the body, inflammation can be identified by redness, swelling, heat to the touch and pain. This can happen when there is an infection, a physical injury or any other assault to that area.

There are many diseases that come about as a result of prolonged inflammation. These diseases are called Inflammatory Diseases. When inflammation occurs for a long period of time, it goes from being beneficial to cause issues for the person's body. Chronic inflammation can occur because of consistent exposure over a long period to a low level of an irritant like allergens or chemicals. When inflammation becomes chronic, we begin to see diseases develop.

Autophagy plays a role in reducing inflammation, especially in the brain. Since autophagy has the ability to both keep cells alive and to cause their death, it can control the presence of inflammatory cells and control their exit when the irritant has been removed. By inducing Autophagy in your body through eating according to the Keto diet, you are able to reduce inflammation by having the inflammatory cells be broken down and removed from the site of the body that they are affecting. Some examples of inflammatory diseases are below;

- Allergies

Allergies to something like a cat when you visit someone's house can come about quickly when in the presence of the cat and be gone after a few days once the irritant is removed. Sometimes, however, the inflammation caused by allergies can become chronic and can lead to a condition like hay fever. This is when the nasal pathways become inflamed in an effort to protect the person from inhaling any more of the irritant (like pollen or grass) however, after a few weeks, this inflammation can become quite irritating to the person experiencing it. They will experience things like a stuffed nose which can make it difficult for the person to go about their regular lives. At this point, inflammation that is supposed to help the person becomes more of a burden.

- Asthma

Asthma is a disease that is caused by inflammation of the tubes that connect and move air to and from the lungs, as well as the tubes within the lungs. Because these airways are inflamed, they are extra sensitive to everything that the lungs inhale, especially irritants of any sort. When an irritant is inhaled, the already inflamed airways become even more swollen which makes it very difficult for the person to breathe. Asthma and allergies are closely linked and can act in similar ways or in tandem in the body. Similar to allergies, chronic inflammation can be caused by environmental factors such as pollution in the air or chronic mold exposure.

- IBD and IBS

Inflammatory Bowel Disease, or IBD, is another disease caused by chronic inflammation, and within the term Inflammatory bowel disease (IBD) there are a number of more specific conditions, all characterized by the inflammation of the digestive tract. IBD is caused by an abnormal response in the gut to certain foods, or bacteria and viruses, leading to chronic inflammation. There are many symptoms that the inflammation of the digestive tract can cause, including nausea, lack of appetite, fever and fatigue as well as abnormal stools. One example of an IBD is Crohn's Disease, where any part of the digestive tract can be the site of inflammation. The food that a person puts in their body is very important when they have IBD, as the food will have to go through the digestive tract and thus, the inflamed areas will be involved every time the person ingests food.

Now that you understand how the above inflammatory diseases happen, you can begin to understand how eating according to a Ketogenic diet can help to improve them, as they are all associated with inflammation. They can all be improved by the presence of autophagy. Autophagy can remedy and reduce the occurrence of these diseases if it is induced at the right times and in the right way. This is why educating yourself about the Plant-Based Ketogenic diet is so important to not only your weight but your health overall.

Autophagy Helps With Many Diseases

Autophagy helps prevent numerous diseases but it also helps those who have existing diseases like cancer, Alzheimer's, and dementia.

Cancer

Cancer is another umbrella term that includes the entire body. There are numerous types of cancers, but they are all based on the same type of dysfunction of the body's cells. Cancer is caused by malfunctions in the growth of cells, either the uncontrolled growth of new cells or the dramatic slowing of the growth of new cells. Sometimes, this rapid increase in cell creation can cause a tumor, but not all cancers involve tumors. Cell death is a normal part of the body's functioning, but sometimes this cell death is not properly executed or communicated. Then, as a result, the cells that are meant to die off and be replaced by new ones do not begin the process of cell death. Because of this, there is a large buildup of cells that begin stealing the nutrients and energy from the other cells that were meant to take their place and the body begins to experience impaired immune function. This also often leads to cancer.

Autophagy can actually reduce a person's risk of cancer. This is because of the way that it is able to clear the body of damaged cells. When damaged cells multiply and divide, this can cause a buildup that can become dangerous and eventually cancerous. If autophagy is functioning properly, it should be able to break down these cells before they can build up, and in this way, autophagy keeps a person healthy and cancer-free. It is for this reason that many people are choosing to take this into their own hands and trigger autophagy within their cells by following a Ketogenic diet.

In addition to triggering Autophagy in your body, there are many ways that you can help to reduce your risk of Cancer through dietary means. We briefly discussed some of these in previous chapters of this book, and here we will revisit them in more depth.

There are many bioactive compounds in food that can reduce your risk of developing cancer. These compounds are things like the following;

- Antioxidants- get rid of harmful by-products produced by

damaged cells, clearing out the harmful clutter and debris in the body.

- 6-Shogaol- Found in ginger and is known to be anti-inflammatory, pain-relieving and nausea-reducing.
- Phytochemicals- Chemicals found in plants that act positively in the body to produce health benefits. Found in vegetables.

These cancer-fighting compounds can be found in plant-based whole foods like Garlic, Ginger, Carrots, Broccoli, tomatoes, dark chocolate, green tea, and so on. This is why eating a plant-based diet is so beneficial for reducing your risk of developing cancer.

Dementia and Alzheimer's

Dementia is a blanket term for a combination of symptoms of cognitive decline such as forgetfulness and disorientation. Alzheimer's disease is one common example of dementia. One cause of dementia is cell death, which we know by now involves autophagy. This brain cell death happens over a period of time and includes gradual cognitive decline as this happens. The actual causes of dementia including Alzheimer's, are not well known, but what is known is that this steady decline is linked to abnormal cell death. Autophagy is signaled to begin in specific cells when there is a programmed cell death that is scheduled to take place. This is so that new cells can be created to take their place. Sometimes though, as in the case of dementia, cell death occurs similarly to in an autoimmune disorder when it is unprogrammed and unwarranted. When this happens in the brain, the results are quite damaging. This is the opposite of cancer when the programmed cell death malfunctions and the cells that are meant to die do not.

There are some foods that you should include in your diet if you want to reduce your risk of developing Alzheimer's disease. These foods contain brain cell-preserving compounds which help to keep the brain cells healthy and reduce the chances of dementia. Some of these compounds and foods that they can be found in are listed below;

- Omega 3 Fatty Acids- Improve cognitive function and reduce inflammation in the brain
- Brussels sprouts, cabbage, Kale – Sulforaphane which is a dementia-slowing phytochemical that acts by protecting the brain cells
- Coffee and the Coffee Cherry- caffeine and antioxidants that are beneficial for brain health
- Green Tea- helps with memory and learning
- Coconut oil- increases Ketosis in the brain leading to better brain health
- Reishi Mushrooms- improve immune function, brain function
- Turmeric- protects the brain cells from damage
- Extra Virgin olive Oil- slows the progression of Alzheimer's

These foods can and should all be ingested regularly when following a Ketogenic diet in order to prevent Dementia and Alzheimer's.

CALCULATING YOUR PERSONAL INTAKE

IF YOU THOUGHT you left math class behind in high school, think again! In this chapter, we are going to look at how to calculate your own personal daily intake of your macronutrients. Macronutrients are those nutrients that are comprised of other smaller nutrients. These macronutrients are carbohydrates, protein, and fat. These are the things that you will often hear about when talking about a food's content and its level of "healthiness."

Why This Calculation Is Important

It is important to get an idea of what your own personal amount of calories, as well as fat and protein intake, should be so that you can determine if you are eating enough, too much or just the right amount. This is helpful when it comes to weight loss. Remember is an earlier chapter when we discussed weight loss and how a calorie deficit is needed to achieve weight loss? This is where we revisit that concept again. If you determine your regular daily intake, this tells you the number of calories that you would need to eat in order to maintain your weight exactly where it is currently. Then, in order to lose weight, you will reduce this number of calories slightly and you will put yourself in a calorie deficit each day, resulting in weight loss over time. You do not need to severely restrict your calories in order to do this, only to have a small deficit and this will lead you to lose weight over time.

*T*his calculation is based on age, sex, height, weight, and activity level, as all of these factors influence your body's use of calories and each macronutrient in particular.

*T*o begin, you will need to calculate your BMR or Basal Metabolic Rate. This is an indicator of the number of calories your body needs in order to simply live. This includes breathing, talking, moving, and so on, without any exercise. The bigger the person's body, the more calories they will need to maintain life. The reason that this calculation takes age into consideration is that as we get older, our amount of muscle generally decreases. Thus, we must take this into account as this reduces the amount of calories needed to run our body's functions. Further, there is a different calculation for men than for women, as male bodies and female bodies use energy differently. You can see these equations below. Plug in your own numbers to get your personal BMR.

· · ·

*B*MR (Basal Metabolic Rate) Calculation for Men

66+ (6.2 x weight in pounds) + (12.7 x Height in inches) – (6.76 x Age) = BMR

*B*MR (Basal Metabolic Rate) Calculation for Women

655.1 + (4.35 x weight in pounds) + (4.7 x Height in inches) – (4.7 x Age) = BMR

*T*he next factor that will go into calculating your macronutrients is to determine your TDEE or your Total Daily Energy Expenditure. This number will tell you how much energy your body uses on a daily basis, including your exercise. While BMR tells you how much energy you use if you were to just live for a day without spending any extra energy, TDEE will give you a more realistic number as it will include your level of activity.

1.2 little to none

1.375 1-3 days of light exercise

1.55 3-5 Days of moderate exercise

1.725 6-7 Days of Hard exercise

1.9 Very intense

*T*o determine your level of activity, you can include everything you do during a regular day that includes more strenuous activity than just sitting, standing or regular walking. Depending on your job, this could be included in your level of activity, such as if you are on your feet all day or if you lift heavy objects.

*T*otal Daily Energy Expenditure (TDEE) Calculation for both women and men;

BMR x (your personal levels of exercise) = TDEE

*T*his number will give you a better idea of the number of calories your body uses in a day, and we will look at how you can adjust this to determine the number of calories you should eat in order to lose weight shortly.

*B*ody Fat Percentage

This step is a little difficult to determine since you need some method of calculation in order to determine it. Your body fat percentage is a more accurate way to determine your weight than stepping on a scale since it will break down for you the percentage of your body weight that is made up of fat. This will help you to determine the amount of weight you want to lose and what a healthy amount of weight would be for your body to lose. Knowing this also will help to determine how much protein you need to intake in order to maintain your muscles. There are multiple ways to determine your body fat percentage.

1. Skinfold Caliper

*T*his is the most common method of measuring body fat percentage. This involves taking measurements of the extra skin on your body. This tool pinches your skin and determines the amount of fat layer that you have in different areas of the body in order to determine an overall percentage.

1. Measuring Tape

*Y*ou can also measure body fat percentage with a measuring tape. You would take measurements of your hips, neck and waist and would then be able to determine your body composition, including the fat percentage. This method gives a more general idea than some of the other methods which tend to be more accurate.

1. X-Ray Scan

*I*f you have access to this at your doctor's office or a clinic of some sort, you can measure your body fat percentage with this special type of X-ray called a DEXA scan. This is the most accurate but the most difficult to get your hands on. It measures your bone density and uses this to determine your body fat percentage for you.

1. Body Fat Percentage Scale

*T*here is a scale that can give you more specific readings than a classic bodyweight measurement scale. This scale is called a Tanita scale. Some gyms or doctor's clinics will have these. When you step on it, it measures your total body weight, your fat percentage and even your water content. This is able to give you a pretty accurate read of your body composition.

1. Visually Estimating

*I*f the other methods are not accessible to you, you can visually estimate your body fat percentage. This would give you the most general and least specific idea, but would help you to get an idea nonetheless. You would examine your body in order to determine how much fat you have versus muscle. Keep in mind that some of your body weight will include ingested water.

*L*ean Body Mass Calculation

Once you know your body fat percentage by using one of the previously mentioned methods, you can determine your lean body mass. This calculation will use your body fat percentage and your total weight to determine your fat by weight, and then a second calculation will use this to determine your lean body mass, which is essentially your body weight minus your fat mass. The calculation is below.

*B*ody fat mass (lbs) = Total weight x body fat percentage as a decimal

*L*ean body mass (lbs) = Total bodyweight – fat mass in pounds

. . .

These two calculations will help you determine how much protein you need to consume in order to maintain your lean body mass. We will look at how to do that later on in this chapter.

Caloric Deficit and Why You Need This

Now that you know how many calories you burn on a daily basis, you can adjust this amount in order to put yourself in a caloric deficit, which will lead to weight loss. If you want to maintain your weight, you will eat exactly as many calories as you need in order to sustain your life and activity level (TDEE). If, however, you want to lose weight, this is what you will do. In order to begin losing weight, the recommended caloric reduction is between 10 and 20%. It is not advised to reduce your caloric intake by any more than 30%, as this can leave you without enough energy to sustain your regular activity and daily life. In order to get the number of calories you should eat in order to lose weight you will do the following calculation;

Calorie Intake for Weight Loss = 10% reduction in TDEE

= 0.1 x TDEE

If you were looking to reduce your calories by 20%, you would do the same equation, but substitute 0.1 for 0.2 instead. Then, you will take this number and subtract it from your

TDEE. An example of this can be seen in the Sample Calculations section below.

Carbohydrate Intake

As we discussed in an earlier chapter of this book, when determining your carbohydrate intake, it is important to look at your actual useable carbohydrates, which is equal to your total carbohydrate intake minus your fiber intake. This is because your body cannot get carbohydrates from fiber. In order to determine your carbohydrate intake on a Plant-Based ketogenic diet, in particular, you will use the following equation;

$$\frac{TDEE \times (\% \text{ of calories})}{4} = \text{Grams of carbohydrates per day}$$

$$\frac{TDEE \times (0.05)}{4} = \text{Grams of carbohydrates, 5\% of daily calorie intake}$$

$$\frac{TDEE \times (0.1)}{4} = \text{Grams of carbohydrates, 10\% of daily calorie intake}$$

· · ·

*F*or this calculation, be sure to use your TDEE that you took ten percent off of, as we calculated in the previous step so that you are determining your carbohydrate intake based on your caloric deficit. Because the ketogenic diet includes between 5 and 10 percent carbohydrates, we will determine a range. We will do this calculation using both 0.05 and 0.1 substituted for percentage in order to determine your carbohydrate range.

*P*rotein Intake

*P*rotein will be about 20-25% of your intake on the Keto diet. As you know now, this number will be determined by your body fat composition, or your lean mass content. This is because the amount of protein you will eat will be largely dependent on the amount of muscle you have. This calculation is a little confusing, so read closely.

*F*or those who are sedentary, use the following calculation;

Lean Body Mass in pounds x 0.6 grams of protein = protein intake in grams

Lean Body Mass in pounds x 0.8 grams of protein = protein intake in grams

. . .

*F*or those who are moderately or lightly active, use the following calculation;

Lean Body Mass in pounds x 0.8 grams of protein = protein intake in grams

Lean Body Mass in pounds x 1.0 grams of protein = protein intake in grams

*F*or those who lift weights or who want to gain muscle, use the following;

Lean Body Mass in pounds x 1.0 grams of protein = protein intake in grams

Lean Body Mass in pounds x 1.2 grams of protein = protein intake in grams

*T*hese above calculations will give you a range of protein intake in grams. If you want to determine what this is in calories, you will multiply them by 4.

*P*rotein intake in grams x 4 = Calories from protein

*F*at Intake

. . .

*O*n a Ketogenic diet, the majority of the calories you intake will come from fat. In this section, we will look at our final calculation, how much fat you will need to intake, even when trying to lose weight. Fat will make up 70-80% of your total caloric intake. This will be the easiest calculation, as we already know the carbohydrate and protein intake. The fat intake will depend on the amount of protein you need, which is why these calculations are so personal to your existing body composition and your goals of gaining muscle, losing weight, or both.

*1*00- (Protein Percentage + Carbohydrate Percentage) = Fat percentage

*E*xamples of Calculations

*T*he following calculations are a sample for a woman who is 35, weighs 143lbs, and is 5'6 in height. Her level of daily physical activity includes moderate exercise 3-5 days per week. Her body fat percentage is 26%.

*B*MR = 655.1 + (4.35 x 143) + (4.7 x 66 inches) – (4.7 x 35)

= 655.1 + 622.05 + 310.2 – 164.5

= 1422.85

· · ·

TDEE = BMR x activity level

= 1422.85 x 1.55

= 2205.42 calories

Body Fat Mass = 143 x 0.26

= 37.18 lbs

Lean Body Mass = 143lbs – 37.18 lbs

= 105.82 lbs

Calorie Intake for Weight Loss = 10% reduction in TDEE

= 0.1 x TDEE

= 0.1 x 2205.42

= 220.54 calories = 10% of your TDEE

= TDEE- 220.54 calories

= 2205.42 – 220.54

= 1984.88 calories

Grams of carbohydrates, 5% of daily calorie intake = $\frac{TDEE \times (0.05)}{4}$

. . .

$$= 1 \frac{984.88 \times 0.05}{4}$$

$$= 99.24 / 4$$

$$= 24.81$$

Grams of carbohydrates, 10% of daily calorie intake = $\frac{TDEE \times (0.1)}{4}$

$$= \frac{1984.88 \times 0.1}{4}$$

$$= 198.49 / 4$$

$$= 49.62$$

Therefore, based on our calculations, this person would be able to eat between 25 and 50 grams of carbohydrates per day.

Lean Body Mass in pounds x 0.8 grams of protein = protein intake in grams

105.82 lbs x 0.8 = 84.66 grams

· · ·

84.66 grams x 4 = 338.6 calories from protein

Lean Body Mass in pounds x 1.0 grams of protein = protein intake in grams

105.82 lbs x 1.0 = 105.82 grams

105.82 grams x 4 = 423.28 calories from protein

Fat percentage = 100- (Protein Percentage + Carbohydrate Percentage)

= 100- (25 percent + 10 percent)

= 100- 35

= 65% Fat intake

Fat percentage = 100- (Protein Percentage + Carbohydrate Percentage)

= 100- (20 percent + 5 percent)

= 100- 25

= 75% Fat intake

. . .

*T*he first calculation above is using the upper threshold of protein and carbohydrate intake percentage, and the second uses the lower threshold. Therefore, her fat intake should come from 65-75 percent of her total calorie intake.

1 984.88 x 0.65 = 1290.17 calories

= 65 percent of total calories

*N*umber of grams of fat = 1290.17 / 9

= 143.35 grams

1 984.88 x 0.75 = 1488.66 calories

= 75 percent of total calories

*N*umber of grams of fat = 1488.66 / 9

= 165.41 grams

*T*herefore, this woman should be eating a total of 1985 calories per day with the following macronutrient intake;

9 9- 198 Calories from carbohydrates

338- 423 Calories from protein

1290- 1489 calories from fat

*I*n order to achieve her desired caloric intake and avoid going over, she will need to keep track of her macronutrient intake, since it is a range. Sticking to the lower end of the range will leave her below 1985, and sticking to the upper threshold will leave her somewhere around 2100 calories, so she will need to be mindful. However, this will give her some flexibility in terms of her food choices and her daily meal choices, as long as they stay within these parameters. This will keep her in ketosis and will lead her on the path to losing weight.

SHOPPING ON A KETOGENIC DIET

ONE OF THE most daunting tasks of following a ketogenic diet is how to properly shop for it. If you are an adult, you likely have done numerous grocery shops and have gotten into a habit and routine of getting certain items every time. This is going to change when you take on a new diet. This chapter will teach you how to approach the grocery store and how to choose the right items in order to have a successful ketogenic diet. Let's jump right in.

Entering the Store With a List

The first thing to keep in mind when grocery shopping for a new diet is to enter with a list. By doing this, you are going to give yourself a guide and this will prevent you from picking up whatever you crave or whatever you feel like eating at that moment. IF you treat it like a treasure hunt, you will be able to cross things off of the list one at a time without venturing to the parts of the grocery store that you do not need to go in and that will simply prove to be a challenge for you to avoid.

Choosing the Meat and Vegetables That You Love

Since the only things that you need to stick to low-carbohydrate foods and meals, you can allow yourself some room for creativity within your shopping experience. If you prefer broccoli over tomatoes, buy broccoli and find new and fun recipes to use broccoli. If you don't enjoy eggplant, you don't have to eat eggplant at all. By giving yourself some creative freedom within the parameters of your diet, you will be able to let yourself feel like you still have choice and control over what you eat, which will help you stick to the diet and avoid feelings of an uncontrolled life which can lead you to abandon the diet quite quickly.

Shop Temptation Free

Since a ketogenic diet is high in fat and proteins, stick to the butcher and meat areas of your grocery store. Avoid the middle aisles, where it is full of carbohydrates and sugars. If you are eating plant-based, you will be spending most of your time in the grocery store around the outer perimeter. This is where the whole, plant-based foods are located. By doing this, and entering with a list, as I mentioned, you will be able to avoid the middle aisles where the processed and high-carb, high-sugar foods are all kept. This will keep you away from temptations and away from foods that you are not going to be eating on this diet.

Do Not Shop When You Are Hungry

One of the biggest things that I mention to everyone when beginning the keto diet is to shop when you are hungry. This will make you reach for anything and everything that you see. By entering the grocery store when you are full or when you have just eaten, you will be able to stick to your list and avoid falling prey to temptations. Make sure you've had a satisfying meal before heading to the grocery store to avoid temptation buys.

EASY KETOGENIC RECIPES AND MEAL PLANS

~~~

IN THIS CHAPTER, I will provide you with a 7-day meal plan that is easy for all beginner keto dieters. This will help you get into the swing of things and for you to have recipes to lean back on when you are in a hurry or don't have time to do additional shopping.

Day 1

Breakfast:

Spinach, mushroom, and feta omelet with keto coffee (coffee with adding fat such as MCT oil, butter, or bone broth protein). "This breakfast is a good source of protein and healthy fats that will keep you feeling full to curb midmorning cravings,"

. . .

*L*unch:

Oven-baked salmon with broccoli. "This lunch features salmon, which is high in heart-healthy fats, as well as broccoli, which is low in carbs but high in fiber," says Dr. Axe.

*D*inner:

Chicken Caesar salad- chicken breast and romaine lettuce, parmesan, and some bacon.

A chicken Caesar salad is a great go-to as it is full of protein and will be just as filling as you need at dinner, this is the perfect meal to finish off your day with!

*Y*ou can also add some olive oil to your dressing to pump up the fat content, as well as plenty of cheese of any type you wish.

*B*onus: Snack

Bacon, Lettuce, Tomato rolls using turkey and avocado.

The BLT is a classic, and by adding turkey and avocado too, it is full of protein, fat and is virtually carb-free, perfect for your new plant-based keto diet.

*I*f you are feeling hungry during the day in response to a lack of carbohydrates, practice eating snacks like this one so that you stay on track and fill your stomach with delicious nutrients like these.

. . .

Day 2
Breakfast:

Whole milk, unsweetened yogurt with a mix of full-fat sour cream, some berries such as strawberries, raspberries, and some seeds like flax seeds and chia seeds, and nuts like sliced almonds and walnuts. When preparing this breakfast, be sure to be mindful of your carbohydrates and your portion size, counting your macros the whole time. This is because all yogurt contains lactose, which technically is counted as a carbohydrate

Pair this parfait with a protein that contains no carbohydrates such as two eggs, and this will help you to get all of your macros in the right amounts.

Lunch:

A healthy lunch-time salad with avocado, nitrate-free, sugar-free bacon, cheese, grape tomatoes, and a variety of nuts and seeds like spicy pumpkin seeds. Add a sugar-free, low-carb, high-fat ketogenic and plant-based salad dressing on top such as ranch or blue cheese dressing, or make your own with olive oil and garlic.

Dinner:

Grass-fed ground beef cooked with onions and a home-made low-carb, no sugar added tomato sauce. Served alongside some grilled zucchini or eggplant, or with carb-free shirataki noodles.

If you need to get your fat intake higher in this meal, if you have not hit your macros for the day, you can sauté your zucchini in olive oil instead of grilling it, or add some extra olive oil infused with garlic directly into your sauce."

Day 3

Breakfast:

A no sugar added full fat Greek yogurt bowl with seeds, nuts, and berries.

Coffee with 2 Tbsp Heavy Cream or half and half (120 calories, 12g fat, 1g net carbs, 0g protein)

Lunch:

Keto lunch box, including sliced grilled chicken, organic, nitrate-free, sugar-free lunch meat such as turkey, any type of cheese cubes that you wish, pickles, a hard-boiled egg, a raw tomatoes, raw vegetables such as cauliflower, carrots, radishes or broccoli, nuts for protein and fat such as walnuts, or almonds, homemade guacamole (avocado, onion, garlic, jalapeno), and no sugar added ranch dressing.

Dinner:

Grilled chicken with a side of grilled eggplant and grilled zucchini as well as cherry tomatoes sautéed in extra virgin olive oil with garlic. By incorporating extra fats with oils or sauces helps to get your fat intake high. This can also be done by including things like coconut cream or heavy cream, to keep you on track.

*D*ay 4

*B*reakfast:

Homemade Sausage & Spinach Frittata, including any vegetables that you wish such as bell peppers, onion, mushrooms, and soon. (206 calories, 16g fat, 1g net carbs, 12g protein)

Coffee with 2 Tbsp Heavy Cream or half and half (120 calories, 12g fat, 1g net carbs, 0g protein)

*L*unch:

Cream cheese with cucumber slices for dipping.

(Cucumber is a low-carb and high-water content vegetable that is versatile and great for a plant-based keto diet)

Hard boiled egg

Keto friendly meatballs

*D*ay 5

. . .

Breakfast:

1/2 cup Ketogenic Egg Salad(166 calories, 14g fat, 1g net carbs, 10g protein) with Romaine Lettuce Wraps (4 calories, 0g fat, 0g net carbs, 0g protein) and 2 slices of cooked bacon diced. (92 calories, 7g fat, 0g net carbs, 6g protein

Lunch:

Homemade guacamole (avocado, onion, garlic, jalapeno, lime juice) with raw zucchini slices for dipping.

Hard boiled egg

Tuna

Dinner:

6 oz of a Rotisserie Chicken (276 calories, 11g fat, 0g net carbs, 42g protein)

3/4 cup cauliflower gratin (cheese, cauliflower, onion, garlic and so on) (215 calories, 19g fat, 2g net carbs, 6g protein)

As well as 2 cups chopped romaine lettuce (16 calories, 0g fat, 1g net carbs, 1g protein) drizzled with 2 Tbsp Caesar Salad Dressing (sugar free) (170 calories, 18g fat, 2g net carbs

Day 6

Breakfast:

Coffee with 2 Tbsp Heavy Cream or half and half (120 calories, 12g fat, 1g net carbs, 0g protein)

5 sticks of celery dipped in 2 Tbsp of peanut or Almond Butter (200 calories, 16g fat, 2.5g net carbs, 7g protein)

Lunch:

2 cups chopped romaine lettuce (16 calories, 0g fat, 1g net carbs, 1g protein) with

2 Tbsp Caesar Salad Dressing (sugar free) to make a small salad(170 calories, 18g fat, 2g net carbs, 1g protein)

1 cup chopped chicken (can use the chicken from the night before) (276 calories, 11g fat, 0g net carbs, 42g protein)

*D*inner:

1 Italian sausage (230 calories, 18g fat, 1g net carbs, 13g protein) with,

1 cup of cooked or raw broccoli (55 calories, 0g fat, 6g net carbs, 4g protein)

1 Tbsp butter that can be added to the broccoli for taste (102 calories, 12g fat, 0g net carbs, 0g protein)

2 Tbsp grated parmesan cheese that can also be added to the broccoli (42 calories, 3g fat, 0g net carbs, 4g protein

*D*ay 7

Breakfast:

2 Keto pancakes, as seen in the recipe chapter above (172 calories, 14g fat, 1g net carbs, 8g protein)

2 pcs cooked bacon (92 calories, 7g fat, 0g net carbs, 6g protein)

Black Coffee with 2 Tbsp Heavy Cream or half and half (heavy cream preferred)

(120 calories, 12g fat, 1g net carbs, 0g protein)

Lunch:

1/2 cup Cauliflower "Pasta" Salad (102 calories, 8g fat, 4g net carbs, 3g protein)

Feta and Sundried Tomato Meatballs (356 calories, 32g fat, 2.5g net carbs, 24g protein)

2 Cups raw baby spinach (14 calories, 0g fat, 1g net carbs, 2g protein)

Spinach can be included in the meatballs or eaten separately

*D*inner:
1 1/2 cups Spicy Spaghetti Squash Casserole

(284 calories, 20g fat, 6g net carbs, 23g protein)

2 cups of baby spinach, raw or cooked with 1 Tbsp ranch dressing (sugar free) drizzled.

Spinach: (14 calories, 0g fat, 1g net carbs, 2g protein)

Dressing (70 calories, 7g fat, 1g net carbs, 0g protein)

Two Bonus Recipes!

. . .

*H*ere are two additional bonus recipes that serve you a delicious keto meal!

Creamy Zucchini Noodle Pasta

Nutritional Information:

1 serving- half of recipe

Calories: 362

Carbohydrates: 16g

Fiber: 9.1g

Fat: 6.3g

Protein: 4.6g

10 mins: Preparation time

5 mins: Cook time

15 mins: Total

Ingredients:

- Water- if and as you need it
- Lemon juice- 1 tablespoon
- Zucchini- 3, cut to strips of ¼ inch width

- Garlic- 1 clove
- Avocado-1
- Fresh basil- ½ cup
- Salt and pepper for tasting
- Olive oil- 2 tablespoons

*I*nstructions:

1. In order for you to make this sauce- combine by placing into a food processor, the avocado, basil leaves, garlic, and lemon juice, and blend this mixture until it becomes smooth.
2. Next, add the extra virgin olive oil and blend again until incorporated.
3. Add some water, 1 Tablespoon at a time just until the sauce becomes fluid but yet still thick in its consistency.
4. Season this sauce with pepper and salt, to taste.
5. To make the Zucchini Noodles if you have never made them before: use a spiral machine or slice them into thin, noodle-shaped strips.
6. Once you have made your noodles, sauté them in a small amount of olive oil on medium to medium-high temperature until they become softer and a brighter green hue. This will usually take about 4 minutes.
7. Drain out the extra water from the pan, and you are ready to serve.
8. To Serve: Toss your zucchini noodles in the sauce you made and add some parmesan cheese to the top.

9. (you will likely have some sauce for leftovers, depending on how many macros you are looking to take in).

The Ultimate Keto Turkey Dinner

Are you afraid that you have to miss out on your traditional turkey dinner this thanksgiving?

Think again!

When following a plant-based, ketogenic diet, you can still experience the joys of a full, hearty, and prize-winning turkey, chock full of flavor and protein!

While I know you love the classic turkey dinner, we are going to look at a way to make an even more delicious, but still keto-friendly turkey dinner. As a bonus, this one also cooks faster and is just about as complicated as a regular turkey dinner is to make. But you get that extra flavor out of it!

Now, this is a little more technical than some other recipes, but it is well worth it. To give you a preview, it is a brined, roasted turkey that is also wrapped in bacon and has a gravy to go with it all. You won't even miss the potatoes you won't be having on this diet.

While in truth, it doesn't lead to the full turkey being roasted in the end, it does lead to a sliced and juicy spread of turkey and bacon, what could be better?

. . .

*Y*ou will wow and impress all of the family this Thanksgiving and you won't even have to answer pesky questions about why you are on a diet that doesn't include the festive meal.

*I*t will be presented already carved and presented on a platter for everyone to devour, and you won't have to fiddle with the knife at the table.

*T*he one recurring issue every thanksgiving is how to keep that turkey from getting dry! This recipe will solve that issue for you. The secret, the brine! The brine is the best kept secret. It works by helping the turkey to absorb the moisture while you leave it brining overnight, and then this will lead to a fatter, juicier turkey than you have ever seen before. Its weight will increase by a whopping 8%, just because of this simple but beautiful secret technique.

Further, as you now know quite a deal about raw versus cooked food, when you brine the turkey overnight, this leads to some of the proteins within the meat to liquify, and some of them to become denatured, which leads to more liquid, more moisture, and more flavor.

*B*efore you begin, be sure you are ready with several large pots and a roasting pan, ice, and a good working thermometer. You want to ensure the turkey is cooked to the perfect point! Not over and not under.

. . .

*H*ere are some extra tips for your turkey dinner:

*F*at is your friend! By rubbing fat (such as butter or olive oil) under the skin of your turkey, this will help to add extra fat which we know is keto's friend.

*D*efrost it! A fresh and defrosted turkey will always be easier to work with. When doing this, to ensure safety, defrost it in your fridge on a plate slowly and let it happen on its own; don't try to speed up the process. Safety is key when it comes to poultry!

*S*maller is better. While it may be tempting to go bigger, having two small turkeys will lead to a better overall cook and more ability to monitor and control the process. Smaller is better!

*R*emoving the bones! It can be quite difficult to learn how to remove the bones, but stick with this one. Watch a few videos to follow along with as you do this; there is no way but to try it. There are a multitude of different ways that this can be done. You will eventually find your own approach and this will be the one you show your kids someday.

. . .

When it comes to tying the roast, it is similar to the point above about removing the bones, stick with it, and be patient, watch some videos if you need to. This will take practice.

This recipe is based on the fact that you are working with a full turkey that has the bones in, which is then split 4 ways- with two thighs with the leg meat still on and two breasts. It is also based on the fact that you have the bones from this turkey as well, in order to make broth and gravy. If you want to go a different route, but these pieces of meat with the bones in and it will still work for you just fine.

Nutritional Information:

Serving size: 12g

Calories: 728.67 calories

Carbohydrates: 1.488g

Protein: 87.49g

Fat: 38.88g

Fiber: 0.244g

1 hour: Prep Time

1 hour, 30 minutes: Cook Time

Total Time

Servings: 12 Servings

Ingredients:

- Turkey, including bones- 20lbs, 1 whole
- Tapioca flour- 1 tablespoon
- pepper and salt to taste
- Twine
- Ice cubes- 4 cups
- Natural sugar replacement- 1 teaspoon
- Onions, chopped- 3
- Kosher salt- ½ cup
- xanthan gum- ½ teaspoon
- Celery cut into pieces- 4 stalks
- Sage- 1 bunch
- coarsely cracked black pepper divided- 1 ½ tablespoon
- Carrots cut into pieces, 4 carrots
- Water, divided- 2 gallons
- Fresh thyme leaves, chopped- 1 tablespoon
- Liquid fat in the form of ghee, bacon fat, or olive oil- ¼ cup
- Garlic cloves, crushed- 8
- Bay leaves- 3

*I*nstructions:

1. The day before Thanksgiving, or whenever you are going to serve this turkey, you are going to get your turkey ready. Remove the bones and keep them aside.

2. Pre-heat your oven to 350 degrees Fahrenheit
3. Grease your roasting pan using whatever fat source you have chosen. Further, cover your turkey bones and the neck with 2 tablespoons of the fat. Put your bones on your roasting pan and put it into the preheated oven. This step is so that the turkey stock will have a more roasted taste.
4. Leave to roast for 30 minutes.
5. After 30 minutes has passed, flip them over and roast the other side for thirty more minutes. Check on them. They should have a golden, roasted color. If they are pale still, flip them once again and roast them for 20 more minutes. Keep going in this way, until they golden brown. (you don't want to get them too dark, in order to avoid having a bitter taste).
6. Once the bones are done, take them out of the oven and put them into another big sized pot with a capacity of at least 2 gallons. Pour your water into the pot, enough to cover them. Depending on the size of your turkey, this will be somewhere around 5.7 L of water.
7. Put the pot on the stove and turn the burner onto medium heat.
8. Deglaze the pan you used to roast the bones. Put the roasting pan on one or two hot burners, depending on its size, and add 1 cup of water. If you prefer, use white wine. Swirl the water or wine around the pan. Using a spoon, scrape the brown residue off of the bottom of the pan. Swirl to combine it into the liquid. A murky brown liquid will result.
9. Pour this liquid into the pot containing the turkey broth.
10. Once turkey broth starts to simmer, lower the heat.
11. Simmer for 3 hours.

CONCLUSION

Following a Keto meal may be easy for some but difficult for others. Keep in mind that strictly following the foods based on this diet will not do the job. You must take things like caloric intake and caloric deficit into consideration as well when you are trying to lose weight. This will not only help you to achieve your goals of weight loss, but it will help you to reduce your risk of developing numerous diseases and will improve your health overall.

When trying to begin the Keto diet, there are some precautions to keep in mind so that you can ensure you are approaching this diet from the most knowledgeable and safest possible position. Since it involves rapid and drastic changes to your macronutrient intake, your body will be shocked at first, and it may wonder what you are doing to it. Once this period passes though, your body will get used to it and will be able to process the high fat and low carbohydrate diet with ease. In no time, you will be feeling better and will be well on your way to your weight loss goals.

The first thing to keep in mind when fasting or when changing to a new diet is the keto flu. When it comes to the keto diet or a low-carb diet specifically, there is something known as the "Keto Flu" that you may experience. This comes with a list of symptoms that are caused by the body trying to adapt to a diet with a dramatic reduction in carbohydrates. These symptoms include nausea, fatigue, headaches, constipation and intense cravings for sugar.

These symptoms could begin somewhere in the first day or two, and the amount of time that they last can vary from a week to multiple weeks. If you experience this, there are steps you can take to stay healthy and help your body to adapt to this dramatic change in diet.

Ever since it began to become popular in mainstream media, the Ketogenic diet has been recommended, along with some supplements that are targeted to assist with aid weight loss. Below is a list of some of the most effective supplements to take in tandem with a plant-based ketogenic diet. Supplements like MCT Oil, keto protein powders, keto electrolytes, digestive enzymes, omega-3, iron and Vitamin-D has been known to help those on a Keto diet.

After reading this book, the next steps are to begin your calculations for your own personal intake if you have not done that yet. Next, read through the multitude of recipes in this book and determine which ones you want to try first. Go ahead and make yourself a meal plan or use the 7-day meal plan provided in the last chapter of this book. Make yourself a grocery list or use the one provided and rid your house of any and all temptation foods if you can-refined carbohydrates and sugars will be the worst culprits. Then, you will have no choice but to follow the diet when you are cooking at home, and by having your weekly meals planned out for you already, you are setting yourself up for success.

www.ingramcontent.com/pod-product-compliance
Ingram Content Group UK Ltd.
Pitfield, Milton Keynes, MK11 3LW, UK
UKHW021455050126
9908UKWH00021B/284